Black America ?

PO Box 971 • Winnsboro, SC 29180

"The complete Resource for America's Minority Pre-Medical Student"

www.blackamericapress.com

Spring 2007

Greetings. Over the past 75 years, the journey to becoming a physician has remained relatively unchanged:attend college, take the MCAT, attend medical school, and then participate in a medical residency program.

Despite this consistency, what has not remained the same is how the journey is executed. As the health care system modernized so has medical education. New techniques, methods, and processes have been developed. Thus, today's students are receiving their medical education and acquiring their knowledge in ways that would not be possible just a few years ago.

One of the newest innovations is the introduction of the computerized version of the Medical College Admission Test (MCAT) in January 2007. Though the basic structure of the exam remains unchanged, this paperless version has made the exam much more student friendly and will give premedical students across the country greater access to the exam.

I recently had the opportunity to take my American Board of Family Medicine recertification exam. The exam was in the computer based format like the MCAT. Having taken all my previous exams on the paper based format I was skeptical. Upon completion of my exam, I found the computer based format far superior. I would never recommend a return to paper and pencil.

I have prepared this insert into "Becoming a Physician: A Complete and Definitive Resource for Aspiring Minority Students" to ensure that the most current MCAT information and advice is received. Please take the time to read and understand the changes when considering the MCAT exam.

-Eric M. Schlueter, MD-

MCAT Update

Introduction

The introduction of the paperless version of the MCAT is a major achievement. The exam has become student friendly and more accessible. Despite these changes, the format of the exam and the importance of the exam have not changed. Students who want to achieve medical school admissions must take the exam seriously.

The computer based exam will be offered 22 times per year over 19 dates. Exams will be offered monthly from April through September. Some morning and afternoon exam sessions are available. As well, weekday and some Saturday testing sessions are available.

The MCAT Format & Scoring

The introduction of the paperless format has not change the question content. A complete understanding of the material presented in the premedical sciences is still required. A good understanding of the English language is necessary for The MCAT is only written in English.

The MCAT opens with an optional 10 minute tutorial. After the completion of each section (see sections below), examinees can take an optional 10 minute break. The exam day ends with a required 10 minute survey. The total test content time is 4 hours and 20 minutes. With the breaks included, the total test time is 4 hours and 50 minutes.

> 1. **Verbal Reasoning** - (60 minutes) – consists of 40 Questions
> 2. **Physical Sciences** - (70 minutes) – consists of 52 Questions
> 3. **Writing Sample** - (60 minutes) – consists of 2 Questions
> 4. **Biological Sciences** - (70 minutes) – consists of 52 Questions

The scoring of the MCAT has not changed. The writing sample is given a letter grade from J (lowest) to T (highest). The other exam sections are scored from 1 (lowest) to 15 (highest). Examinees will receive their scores in about 30 days after the test is completed. MCAT scores are automatically released to the AMCAS application system.

The Test Centers

Examinees will take the paperless version of the MCAT at Thomson Prometric testing centers. These centers are located in multiple cities in each state. Thus, extensive travel is not required. An extensive list of test center locations can be found on the internet at http://www.aamc.org/students/ mcat/testsites.htm. Each test center is small, offers space for about 16 examinees, and provides a comfortable climate controlled environment. Each examinee will have a private computer workstation with comfortable seating. The stations are separated by dividers which allow greater concentration and fewer distractions. Examinees are not permitted to bring anything into the computer lab other then their clothes and a watch. Lockers are provided for jackets and personal items. Ear plugs are available.

Registration for the MCAT

Six months prior to each test date, online registration will start. Registration will close two weeks prior to each test date. All seats at a test center are held for MCAT examinees until 60 days prior to the test date. After that date, the seats will be released for students who wish to register for other computer based testing that may be offered at that site.

Premedical students may take the MCAT up to three times a year. There is no waiting period between exams. A student may hold only one exam registration at a time. Registration may only be completed online at https://services.aamc.org/20/mcat/.

During registration, students will select a test center location, test date, and test time. Registration requires a social security number, contact number, e-mail address, and payment information.

Examinees may cancel their registration at anytime up to 7 days prior to the exam. However, only a 50% refund will be offered. Students who cancel less than 7 days before the exam or do not show up for the exam will not receive a refund. Once registration is complete, students may go online and change their test date and location. A change in test date or location will result in an extra fee. The AAMC offers a fee assistance program. This assists examinees who without financial assistance would be unable to take the MCAT. Application information may be obtained online at www.aamc.org/fap.

Exam Fees

Regular Registration $210   **Late Registration Fee $60**
Change of Test Center Fee $50   **Change of Date Reschedule Fee$50**

Note: If a date and test center change is made at the same time the fee will only be $50

The AAMC Fee Assistance Program reduces the MCAT cost from $210 to $85

The Test Day

The combination of a shortened MCAT and the paperless version means that the exam day has been shortened by about 30%. No longer is this a whole day affair! Examinees are expected to arrive at the test center at least 30 minutes prior to the start of the exam. Late arrival means forfeiture of the exam and registration fee. All examinees are required to bring one valid and current form of government-issued identification containing both a photo and a signature. A valid and current driver's license or passport is acceptable. Any expired form of identification will not be accepted.

The Test Session

Examinees are expected to be familiar with the use of a keyboard and mouse. During the writing section the examinee is expected to type the essay. Basic typing skills are essential. Word processing options such as edit, cut, paste, and copy are all available. Spell check is not available. On the other test sections, the computer will allow examinees to highlight passages and strike out answer choices. All questions within each section may be reviewed and answers changed at any time. However, once a new section is started, access to completed sections is prohibited.

The computer test sessions are secure. All answers are saved. If technical issues occur, a recovery feature is in place. During the test, examinees may void their test. The test will not be scored. Registration fees will not be refunded.

Strategies for Success

The change in format of the MCAT should not affect a student's strategy for success. As discussed on pages 38 - 39, each student should determine the type of review program that will meet their needs and financial resources. All students should take multiple practice tests. These tests are available at www.e-mcat.com and http://www.aamc.org/students/mcat/practicetests.htm. Examinees should also practice typing writing sample essays in exam like conditions.

The availability of multiple exam times should not lull premedical students into choosing a late exam date. Premedical students who test during April or May will be able to complete their applications early in the application cycle. These applications will be quickly evaluated and interviews granted. Students who choose an exam date in July, August, or September will not be able to submit a timely application. They will be caught in the usual application rush. Students who choose an early test date have the option of retesting in August or September with enough time between exams for review.

The strategies for taking multiple choice exams like the MCAT as outlined on pages 40 - 41 remain true. There is a test taking skill that should be developed by taking multiple practice exams in exam like conditions. The physical and psychological preparation for the MCAT as outlined on pages 42 - 43 remain true except for what you will be required to bring to the exam center.

The dramatic expansion of testing opportunities and ability to take the exam up to three times in a testing cycle can provide a false sense of security. Each premedical student should develop a review program that will produce the best possible score the first time around. Preparing for and taking the MCAT multiple times is very time consuming, stressful, and financially draining.

To remain current on the MCAT visit: http://www.aamc.org/students/mcat/start.htm.

Becoming a Physician

A Complete and Definitive Resource for Aspiring Minority Students

Eric M. Schlueter, MD

Black America Press

In dedication to my shining stars
Marcus Isaiah and Maya Iman Schlueter

Becoming a Physician:
A Complete and Definitive Resource for Aspiring Minority Students

Published by
Black America Press
PO Box 971
Winnsboro, SC 29180

ISBN:-10: 0-9777384-1-8
ISBN:-13: 978-0-9777384-1-0

For information please visit on the web at: **www.blackamericapress.com** or to
contact the author by e-mail send your message to: **author@blackamericapress.com**

Contents At a Glance

Contents At a Glance

Contents At a Glance

Contents At a Glance

Acknowledgements

I n the pre-medical experience most quickly find they are are unable to do it alone. Instead all rely on a number of individuals along the way for advice, criticism, support, guidance, encouragement, and love.

In completing this book, I have relied on many people and have to acknowledge their contributions. First, I have to give all praise to my parents, Al Schlueter and Vianna Biehl. Each of whom has played an instrumental role in seeing me grow from a young toddler into an aspiring man. I also am grateful to my wife, Ina Schlueter, for her love, dedication, and the encouragement to shake the dust off the manuscript and to get it published.

I give thanks to my medical school Case Western Reserve University (CWRU). It was very instrumental in providing me with the original tools that allowed me to document all my pre-medical thoughts and experiences, and most of the historical documentation for this book came from its wonderful historical library. I also give special thanks to the following medical students from the CWRU class of '97: Terrence Wadley, Tracy Peatross, Teresa Myers, Dorthy White, Cedrice Davis, Karana Pollard, and from the class of '98: Delani Mann, Ifeolowa Fadeyi, Adrienne Charles, Alfredmy Chesser and Maria Gracia Galvez Picon. All have provided me with great insight into their pre-medical careers.

The greatest African American medical historian of our time is William Montague Cobb; 1904-1990. He served as Professor and Chairman of the Anatomy Department of Howard University and helped train over 6,000 physicians. As well, he served as editor-in-chief and editor emeritus of the Journal of the National Medical Association from 1949 till his death. Over these years he documented the fascinating story and lives of so many African American physicians and their achievements. Without his work, much of African American medical history would have been lost. And for his efforts, he is an inspiration and I give him thanks.

Lastly, I give thanks to Robert Haynie, M.D., Ph.D. His presence in my life during my medical student years was inspirational. America is in an era were there are few African American physicians in medical academia. The time he took out of his busy schedule to reach out to me and other minority medical students did not go unnoticed. It is my hope that physicians of color in academia adopt his commitment to giving and caring for future minority medical students.

-Eric M. Schlueter, MD-

Introduction

Welcome my fellow pre-medical high school and college students, pre-medical advisors, fellow physician mentors, parents, and all who are interested in the continuing growth and development of the minority physician in the United States.

The creation of a medical doctor often begins very early in life. It is the parental support of creativity, intellectual curiosity, inquisitiveness, assertiveness and the promotion of positive self esteem, security, and love. In elementary school it is the encouragement of reading, writing, grammar, arithmetic, artistry, the sciences, and social learning. In junior high school it is the establishment of adequate learning, study, social development, self motivation, and the social interaction with mentors who have achieved some level of success. In high school it is the solidification of one's educational abilities as a life long learner, real work experiences, and the establishment of independence from family life. Educationally and socially armed, the motivated college student navigates their way into medical school.

Despite the ambitious aspirations of many minority students, the events of life seem to get in the way and the goal becomes unreachable. Though tremendous social progress has been made among America's minority groups, there are still many students who are the first in the family not only to attend college but even consider a medical career. Hometown family and friends are encouraging and supportive but lack the experience to provide accurate advice. And, the public educational system in many predominantly minority communities often are more focused on developing programs for students who are at risk of dropping out of school or have technical career aspirations. Thus, few resources are available to provide adequate pre-medical guidance and support. This trend often continues in college. A student may make poor decisions, get behind, and the goal of becoming a physician disappears from the horizon.

Despite the higher number of minority men and women attending college, we have not seen a large enough increase in students who apply to or graduate from medical school. Statistics from the Association of American Medical Colleges Facts and Figures 2005 show that:

In 1980, there were 2,507 **Black** applicants (1,043 were accepted) and 768 graduates (5.3% of the class)
In 2001, there were 2,887 **Black** applicants (1,203 were accepted)
In 2004, there were 1,034 graduates (6.7% of the class)

In 1980, there were 1,764 **Hispanic** applicants (832 were accepted) and 462 graduates (3.1% of the class)
In 2001, there were 2,178 **Hispanic** applicants (1,076 were accepted)
In 2004, there were 1,007 graduates (6.4% of the class)

In 1980, there were 156 **Native American** applicants (65 were accepted) and 33 graduates (.21% of the class)
In 2001, there were 263 **Native American** applicants (134 were accepted)
In 2004, there were   98 graduates (.62% of the class)

Over the past 24 years there was an increase of only 266 Black, 545 Hispanic, and 65 Native American graduates per year. Based upon these numbers, this country is producing less than 21 Black and Hispanic graduates a year for each state. And even more concerning less than 2 Native American graduates a year for each state.

These numbers are totally unacceptable and grossly inadequate to make an impact on all the vital primary and specialty care needs in the growing minority community. The current graduation rate will never allow the Black, Hispanic, or Native American medical profession to attain a racial composition to that of its population in America. According to the AAMC's "Minorities in Medical Education: Facts and Figures 2005", there are 705,960 physicians and 36,225 or 5.1% are Hispanic, 31,225 or 4.4% are Black, and 1,175 or 0.1% are Native American. Currently 12.5% of our population is Hispanic, 12.3% is Black, and 0.9% is Native American.

With the expansion of America's health care system and non-clinical physician opportunities within this system, the rather stagnant number of minority physicians being produced over the past 24 years may be causing the total percentage of minority physicians actually working in clinical medicine to decline. This is at a time when the demand for primary care and major sub-specialty physicians in minority communities is increasing. The lack of an adequate minority physician supply has left these communities medically underserved. This is a contributing factor to the higher than average morbidity and mortality these communities face.

If our communities are going to survive, there has to be a larger minority physician supply. America's health care system is currently one of the largest employment and economic sectors of our society. With so much money involved, there has to be an effort to see that a proportional amount is being spent and invested in the minority community. Using their influence and position, an increased number of minority physicians can work to ensure that more of this money is spent and invested in ways that will support the community. They can influence such areas as ensuring expanded employment opportunities and promotions to minorities; ensure adequate resources are devoted to patient care; utilize minority owned ancillary medical supply, health care, and technology companies; and ensure that bio medical and clinical research monies are being spent in ways that will benefit the minority community.

With a concern for increasing America's minority physician supply, I have written this guide. It contains a compilation of all the advice I received as a pre-medical high school and college student. I pray this guide will help de-mystify the pre-medical experience.

It is difficult to have great career aspirations if we do not know from where we came. It is very important for all of us to recognize that African Americans, Hispanic Americans, and Native Americans have all played an integral role in providing medical care. We should be proud of the many men and women who came before us and paved the road through their tears and sacrifice. There is no doubt that all of us have earned a right to be involved in every aspect of America's health care system. To this end, after each chapter, I have provided short essays outlining the lives of great minority physicians and some of the events they have been a part of. I expect these essays will encourage you to follow in their footsteps.

In closing, I hope this guide will inspire you to have big dreams, set lofty goals, and work hard. Graduation from High School, College, and Medical school are the ultimate accomplishments on the level of Olympic gold medals, Super Bowl victories, or Platinum selling albums. And you will do it three times over with your three degrees. It is my opinion that all of us have the capability to become successful physicians; we just have to understand the means by which to attain that success. And, as you finish the race, don't forget your personal responsibility of contributing to the success of those that follow you. Let's work together and share what we learn with those that are following in our footsteps. It is through this process that we will survive the adverse conditions we face and continue to strengthen our precious communities.

Chapter I

Medical school is a marathon. If you have the endurance and the stamina you will win the race.
-Eric M. Schlueter, MD-

What is it like to be a Physician?

Our society is fascinated with physicians and the work they do. Television has allowed the public to see some of this work through dramatic programming. However, there is much more to being a physician than is shown on the television screen. The life of the physician is very complex. The actual delivery of medical care is only one component to a physician's life. There are often competing demands and obligations the physician has to juggle including the delivery of medical care, continuing education, professional and social commitments, and family.

To understand the heart of a physician we have to go back in time and look at how most fall in love with the profession. The hallmark of all physicians is first and foremost their love of science, particularly the function of the human body: how food is digested and used as fuel, how a cut on the skin or a broken bone heals itself, the complex functions that occur so a finger can move, how the immune system fights off an infection, etc. The human body is the most complex machine in the world and the scientific advances of the past 200 years have provided us with a detailed understanding of it. Yet, there is still much to explore, discover, and understand. Secondly, most physicians have a keen desire to make a substantial difference in people's lives through public service.

Physicians have the responsibility to take all the scientific knowledge, theory, and understanding to the front lines and apply it to the real world of patient care. This requires being able to assess a patient's complaints, examine the body, put the information together, match it up with a known clinical condition, and ultimately treat the condition with medication, surgery, recommendations of lifestyle changes, etc. All the while, the physician has to be able to explain complicated scientific concepts in an easy and understandable way.

Often the assessment, diagnosis, and treatment cannot be carried out in an easy "cook book" like fashion. Each patient brings a unique set of symptoms, physical exam findings, and social circumstances which require a through assessment and unique treatment plan. This is why we consider medicine to be an "art". What works well for one patient may not work well for another. Physicians in consultation with the patient must determine the treatment plan that will lead to the best possible outcome.

The physician derives great satisfaction from bringing healing and health to a patient with significant disability from a medical problem. The patient is often grateful toward the physician. Thus, over time the patient and physician develop a close, trusting, honest, and personal relationship that can last a lifetime.

The physician is also a social worker and motivational speaker. Some patients come in with numerous complaints that are not due to a serious illness or disease but to personal stress, poor living

Becoming a Physician

conditions, lack of access to medications. Thus, the physician must be able to recognize such situations, ask probing questions, and help the patient find the necessary resources. As well, some patients carry self-destructive behaviors like smoking, drug use, over or under eating, alcohol abuse. It is up to the physician to not only recognize these situations but also use all their power and authority of persuasion to encourage the patient to change their behavior.

On television, physicians are often depicted delivering medical care in the hospital or emergency room. However, a majority of clinical medicine is delivered in an office setting where one or more physicians provide medical services. Usually this is a small business owned by the physician(s). Therefore, as a small business owner, the physician is responsible for managing office finances and expenses as well as make important decisions as: employee hiring and firing, pay scale, vacation time, equipment acquisition, record management, and billing. The amount of revenue is based upon how many hours a physician decides to work, the number of patients seen, and the type of services that are provided. To generate enough revenue, the physician is required to work efficiently and think quickly because as one patient is seen three more are often waiting. In today's volatile market and system of managed care, physicians are often challenged and stressed by the same factors that affect all small businesses.

Many physicians provide medical care in the hospital setting also. However, due to the time constraints, some primary care physicians have chosen not to provide services in the hospital but instead rely on a "Hospitalist" physician whose job is to provide medical services exclusively in the hospital. Most physician specialists and surgeons do not have this option and often are forced to balance their time between work in the office and the hospital.

The delivery of medical care does not fit into the convenient hours of 9:00am and 5:00pm Monday through Friday. People get sick at all hours, and thus medical care has to be available at all hours of the day and night. Many physicians have extended office hours on weekday evenings and some even open their offices on the weekend. As well, all physicians are responsible to provide twenty-four hour healthcare coverage. When the office is closed a physician will be available to answer patient telephone questions, assist the emergency room when a patient needs admission to the hospital, and is responsible for any patient care in the hospital. For some physicians, being "on call" can mean a very stressful and busy night or weekend with little sleep or personal time. Many physicians are "on call" one or two nights a week and at least one weekend a month if not more.

The physician is known as a life-long learner. Medicine is continually advancing with new methods of care, treatment modalities, scientific and technical advances, such that the advances of today quickly become the ancient practices of tomorrow. The physician must keep current to render the best medical care to patients. As a result, physicians often attend educational scientific meetings, read journals, and rely on colleagues for assistance in difficult situations. Fortunately, many of the scientific meetings are conveniently located in places that allow physicians great recreational opportunities for themselves and their families.

The work and responsibility of the physician does not stop here. Physicians often are members of local, state, and national medical societies. As members, they attend meetings and serve in various positions to advance their medical specialty. As members of a hospital medical staff, physicians attend medical staff meetings and participate on hospital committees. As well, some physicians enjoy the scientific nature of the profession and engage in clinical research, write journal articles, and lecture at educational conferences.

The physician's life is often filled with a high level of emotional stress. It can be draining trying to balance hospital, office, educational, and professional duties. Added to this is the physician's role in making important decisions that affect real people on a daily basis. Some of these decisions are made very quickly such as when a patient comes into the emergency room very ill or when a person's heart or breathing unexpectedly stops and resuscitative efforts have to be made. Fortunately, most of these decisions produce health, relieve suffering, and are associated with happy outcomes. However, despite the best efforts, physicians are not able to cure every ailment. In addition, physicians are exposed to patients who experience a significant amount of pain, suffering, and even death. In order to survive, the physician has to learn how to balance being emotionally sensitive and compassionate yet not become incapacitated and unable to perform the job each time a difficult emotional situation arises.

Despite all that goes on in a physician's professional life, the greatest challenge often comes trying to balance the professional life with family life. In the past, the physician's first duty was toward medicine. Because people have needs at any time, the older physicians often saw very little of their families and missed out on important family events and holidays. Today the average physician still works 50 to 80 hours per week just to complete the most basic duties and obligations. However, there is a greater awareness that family life is very important to the overall health of the physician. As a result, the profession is slowly accommodating more reduced or part-time work schedules and becoming family friendly.

One of the benefits of being a physician is the salary. Most full time physicians earn over $100,000 per year and live a financially comfortable life. However, this is not without hard work, considerable personal liability, and responsibility. In addition, the physician does not begin to earn this salary till they have completed all medical training which is often seven to twelve years after completion of college. Thus, this is not a get rich quick profession.

One of the great benefits of being a physician is the opportunity to work late in life. Clinical medicine is a mentally and emotionally taxing. However, it often is not physically demanding. Thus, a physician who learns to pace life, take breaks when needed, and maintains a healthy balance between work and family often can practice medicine beyond the usual retirement age.

Today's medical system is fraught with more paper work, administrative duties, and concerns about malpractice liability. This has overwhelmed some physicians and they will give you a pessimistic view of the profession. However, like other businesses and professions, medicine is continuously changing. Physician are challenged to change along with it. The physicians who are able to accommodate these changes and meet the challenges of the times will succeed and enjoy a very satisfying medical career.

Becoming a Physician

Medicine is a wonderful profession. The physician - patient relationship is not found in many other professions. This is a noble, respected, and selfless profession. The physician is a leader and someone who is admired. No matter how the public views the medical profession, it often overwhelmingly rates their personal physician as one of the most important people in their lives. The physician is often the cornerstone of any community. Serving on civic and business associations, government commissions, and community projects; the physician's input is desired and considered important.

Let this be your introduction to the profession. Meet with your personal physician. Ask questions and get a glimpse of their experience. However, do not stop there. Seek other physicians in your community and begin to formulate your own assessment of this profession. A lot of time and effort is required to become a clinical physician. Know beyond all doubt that this is what you want to do before you invest a significant amount of your life toward achieving this goal.

Character Counts

Thirty or forty year ago, there was never much discussion about the character of the physician. Today it is different. It is becoming very common for medical schools, medical residency programs, and state medical licensing boards to require criminal background checks. Therefore, it is imperative for all students to act responsibly and obey the law. Anything otherwise may be enough to keep you out of clinical medicine regardless of how intelligent you may be.

Sadly, I read of physicians in my state who have their medical license revoked or suspended because of lawlessness or improper interactions with patients. Physicians have been reprimanded for the illegal distribution of controlled substance prescriptions outside of the physician-patient relationship and even personal possession and distribution of narcotic drugs. They also have been found guilty of unethical or unprofessional conduct that is likely to defraud, deceive, or harm the public as it relates to medical record keeping and inappropriate and unprofessional conduct of a sexual nature toward a patient, hospital or office staff. As well, some physicians have become addicted to alcohol and or drugs to such a degree that they are unfit to practice medicine.

I often wonder why someone who has invested so much time, money, and energy would gamble and lose it so quickly. However, these addictions often begin as innocent acts used to help relieve or cope with the stress of college, medical school, residency, or medical practice. Do not fall in this same trap. Work now to develop great character traits and a healthy lifestyle that will last a lifetime.

Medical History Gazette

Vol 1, No 1• The First Source for Medical History •Columbia, S.C.

News Flash!

Imhotep:
The World's First Great Physician

In North East Africa, along the great Nile river, one of the world's greatest civilizations developed. Around 3,100 B.C. the upper and lower Egyptians united establishing the Egyptian dynasty. Today, the Egyptians are known for the pyramids, hieroglyphics, and the practice of mummification. However, it is generally unknown that the Egyptians were renown for their medical system. The system had developed such a high standard, that the famous medical philosopher Hippocrates[1] (the commonly acclaimed "Father of Medicine") went to study in Egypt.

The most famous of the Egyptian physicians was Imhotep[2]. As Prime Minister to the Pharaoh Djoser (2980-2900 B.C. 3rd dynasty), he was a statesman of the first rank; as designer and builder of the world's first great edifice in stone, the step pyramid of Saqqara, he was a brilliant architect; and he was the epitome of the sage. Mastery of any one of these areas would have marked a great man, but Imhotep was recorded to have excelled in all. But, even these extraordinary talents appears to have been overshadowed by his gifts as the earliest known physician.[3]

> Egyptians understood many aspects of anatomy, physiology, and parasitology. As well they routinely performed physical diagnoses, prescribed medicine, and performed surgery.

In 1862 A.D., a papyri[4], which was believed to have been written in 1700 B.C., was discovered in the city of Thebes. Summing the knowledge of Imhotep and his disciples, the document outlined proper diagnosis, prognosis, and treatment of 48 surgical cases involving injuries from the head to the chest and spine.[5] In addition, the brain was described for the first time in recorded history.

Some historians have commented that if the work of Imhotep and his followers had been known before those of Hippocrates and his disciples, the title "father of Medicine" might properly have been considered for Imhotep.[6]

In spite of not receiving this special designation, papyric fragments from the second century A.D. show that Imhotep had become such a well know figure in Egyptian civilization that he was deified and a temple was erected on the island of Philae in his honor.[7]

The system of medicine that Imhotep established allowed his Egyptian successors

See **Imhotep** next page

Imhotep: Continued from previous page

to understand aspects of anatomy, physiology, and parasitology. The Egyptians were routinely performing physical diagnoses and prescribing drugs. Surgery was commonly carried out using knives to remove hair, open abscesses, and to extract tumors.[8] After surgery, the wounds were bandaged with linen dressings.

Today remnants of the Egyptian medical system remain with us. The well-known insignia for prescriptions, Rx, was first used in Egypt. According to Egyptian legend the insignia symbolizes godly protection and recovery.[9] Another well known insignia, the caduceus[10], also has its origins in Egypt.[11] Between 250 B.C. and 400 A.D. the god of healing, Chounbic, was symbolized with a serpent staff. The staff is a symbol of authority and the emblems attached denote under whose sponsorship it is wielded. One of the serpents represents death, evil, and disease. The other serpent represents immortality, eternal youth, wisdom, and healing. The snakes are symbolic of the physician's duty of fighting disease and bringing health.

Medicine in the "New World"

To some, the discovery of the "new world" is about how Europe brought its knowledge, intellect, and socialization to a new people. Rather the opposite is true. The Meso-American Indians (members of the aboriginal people inhabiting Mexico and Central America) established the first medical school and hospital in Mexico around 1523. They had a vast supply of herbal medications to use. Medicines were stored in houses and used for specific afflictions and conditions.

Before the influence of the Spanish in the "new world", Aztec physicians knew and could distinguish illness. They participated in surgery and treated wounds. Bone fractures were set in a plaster cast and strengthened by a splint. The Aztec's ideas on sickness and medicine and their practices were an inextricable mixture of religion, magic and science. Many Aztec medical practices were more effective than that of the early Spanish doctors. These physicians often were sent to study the Aztec medicine and herbal practices.

Like the Meso-American Indians and Aztecs, Native Americans have a rich medical experience. Due to the wide variety of distinct Native American nations, this experience is quite broad and diverse. Health and illness is often based upon the balance one has in the community, the earth, and the universe. The treatment approach is to focus not just on the physical but also the mind and spirit. Each of these areas is so interconnected that successful rejuvenation can not be achieved unless all are promoted.

The treatment of physical, emotional, and spiritual ailments usually combines an extensive knowledge and use of local medicinal plants, spirituality, and magic. Some of today's most popular herbal remedies have been used for centuries by many Native American nations. It is estimated that over 200 medical drugs can be linked to Native Americans for their healing use. Communities traditionally have expert healers sometimes referred to as Medicine Men or Medicine Women.

See **New World** next page

New World: Continued from previous page

Today, Native American healers continue the tradition passed down from each generation. In addition, they provide a very important service. Often they fill a deep void left by modern medicine, which tends to neglect spiritual, emotional, and cultural needs.

Moments and Discoveries in Medical History

1674 Bacteria was first described in Europe.

1733 The first measurement of blood pressure was made.

1735 The first medical society was formed in Massachusetts.

1751 The first permanent general hospital in the United States opened up in Philadelphia.

1764 The first medical college in the United States opened its doors.

1816 The first stethoscope of any kind was introduced.

1845 Ether was first introduced as an anesthesia for human use.

1849 The first woman in the United States was conferred a Doctorate of Medicine degree.

1854 Dr. John V. Degresse became the first Black physician to be admitted to the Massachusetts Medical Society.

1855 Indiana becomes the first state to require physicians to have a medical license.

1861-1865 Eight Black physicians serve as commissioned officers in the Army Medical Corps of the Union army during the civil war.

1876 Meharry Medical College was established.

1892 Viruses were first described.

1895 X-rays are discovered.

1896 Dr. Austin Maurice Curtis an 1891 graduate of Northwestern U. Medical School became the first Black physician to be appointed to the staff of a non-segregated hospital, the surgery department of Cook County Hospital in Chicago.

1899 Aspirin is first introduced by a German company, "Beyer"

1900 The A, B, and O blood types were first discovered.

1906 The EKG was first introduced.

1910 Sickle Cell Anemia was discovered.

1910 There were 3,409 Black Physicians in the United States

1917 Lillian Singleton Dove, a Black woman graduate from Meharry Medical college is regarded as the first Black female surgeon.

1917-1918 There were 365 commissioned Black medical officers who participated in World War I.

1930 The National Institutes of Health was established in Bethesda, Maryland.

1930 The Medical College Admissions Test (MCAT) was developed

1947 There were 79 medical schools in the United States. 25 of them barred the admission of Black Students.

1965 Medicare and Medicaid were developed.

1970 The National Health Service Corps was established.

Chapter II

Pre-Medical Planning: The High School Years

It is never too early to begin planning your pre-medical career. As a high school student work to prepare yourself for college. The main areas to consider are academics, summer programs, and your college selection and application.

Academics

The most important thing in high school is to do as well as you can in your classes. There is nothing that can replace a good academic performance and grade point average. However, rather than just getting all A's and B's, it is important to learn the material. If you do not, you will encounter major obstacles when you take the SAT or ACT exams for entrance into college. These exams test your fundamental knowledge acquired in your high school courses.

In preparing for college level science and math courses, I suggest you take a minimum combination of biology, chemistry, algebra, and physics. The more material you learn and understand, during high school, the better your chances are of being a successful pre-medical college student.

Please note that there will be specific concepts presented in your high school science courses that will be difficult to understand. This happens to all of us when we are given complex material for the first time. Do not despair; many of these complex concepts will be presented again during your college years. The second time around they usually make more sense.

Your science education is similar to learning a language. You can't speak until you learn the words and you can't write sentences until you learn the grammar. Your high school science courses are about learning the words and the grammar. Once you have a foundation in these two areas then you will be able to speak the scientific language and write in a scientific manner.

With this in mind, realize that your college education is based on the knowledge you acquire in high school. Thus, your ability to do well in college is based on how well you understand the material presented to you during high school. Similarly, your ability to understand the material presented in medical school will be based on how well you understand the material presented in your college science and math courses. Ultimately your ability to become an excellent physician will be based on your grasp of the material presented in medical school. Start the process rolling now! Do well in all your high school classes.

Due to the extensive variability in the quality of classroom teaching in high school, the quality of your overall science education may rest upon your shoulders. Seek out your science teachers and let them know you have an interest in science and want to become a physician. When you let them know about your interest they are more likely to provide you with help, encouragement, and extra time when you run into difficulties. Establishing a good relationship with your science teachers will also be a great benefit when it is time for you to apply to college because they can write an excellent letter of recommendation.

Pre-medical students, are expected to excel in their math and science classes. However, if success is truly going to come, you also have to excel in the English classes. English is important because in college and medical school you are expected to read a large volume of material quickly and with full comprehension. In addition, you will be expected to write fluently and articulate your ideas and thoughts. As a future physician, much of your career will depend upon your ability to read, comprehend, and evaluate the many advances in medicine. Also you may be called upon to write scholarly material describing these new advances.

Establishing excellent reading and writing skills does not occur over night. Instead, it takes months and years of practice. Go to the library during your vacations, check out interesting books and read them. As you find words you do not know, look them up in a dictionary. As your vocabulary expands, your writing will improve. You will have a larger pool of words that can be utilized to describe your thoughts. It is important to practice writing in your English classes because you still have to learn how to use your new words (grammar) so your thoughts come out correctly on paper. There is no one better to help you do this than your English teacher.

Many students entering college have poor study habits. As a result, their college experience has a rocky start. Most freshmen realize their study habits in high school just do not work anymore. College professors structure their courses so that more material is covered in a shorter amount of time compared with high school. To prevent yourself from experiencing a rocky beginning in college, establish a good study pattern today! Establishing good study habits does not occur overnight but takes time, effort, and the determination to seek improvement. To begin establishing good study habits read the section "Enhancing your study techniques" in chapter III. If you can adopt this program, you will be on the road to a successful academic career.

Summer Programs

Summer programs provide an opportunity to gain medical or research experience. It is important to have exposure to the medical field as early as possible. The exposure you receive will help you understand what medicine is like and whether it is a suitable career for you. At this point in your education it is not important to try and figure out what type of physician you want to become. Deciding that you want to become a physician is a great first step.

If there is a medical school in your area, contact the school's admissions or minority affairs office and ask if they offer any summer programs for high school students. If there is not a medical school or it does not offer a summer program, stop by your high school's guidance counselor and ask if a local college / university or hospital sponsors a medical oriented summer program. If the counselor is not available, you can contact a local hospital or college admissions office and they can direct you further. Do not forget about your local physicians or nursing homes. Feel free to call and ask to speak to the office manager or nursing home director. Inform them of your interest of becoming a physician and desire to shadow their physician(s) or volunteer in the home. Often, physicians and nursing home staff are willing to help a student who demonstrates an active interest in medicine. Lastly, consider contacting your state's Area Health Education Center (AHEC). These centers often offer health career enhancement and recruitment programs for minority high school students. Visit http://bhpr.hrsa.gov/ahec/ for more information.

In the event you are not able to participate in a medically oriented summer program, pursue a summer research project with one of your science teachers or have one of them refer you to a project going on at a local college or university. Participating in scientific research can boost your academic ability because you will gain new scientific knowledge and you might be able to receive more individual attention than your high school teacher is able to provide in the classroom.

In addition to the knowledge and experience summer programs provide, you will also gain something substantial to write down on your college application(s). Besides grades and test scores, many competitive colleges and universities look for experiences that make a student stand out relative to the rest of the applicant pool. Participation in summer programs will definitely make you stand out.

Summer is often a time for high school students to earn extra money for personal expenses. In addition, the desire and pressure to fulfill this need often can be very intense: especially when trying to keep up with classmates. However, many summer programs provide their participants with a stipend. This great feature that allows students to participate and still earn some personal spending money.

Applying to College

One of the most important tasks in your educational career is applying to college. This task can seem overwhelming, so begin early. During your freshman and sophomore years, speak to students who graduated from your high school and are in college. Listen to their success stories and pitfalls. Determine if any of these schools are places you want to attend.

In your junior year, you should begin to make a list of the colleges you want to attend. Examples include historically black colleges, rural or urban colleges, large universities or small colleges, public or private colleges, very competitive or moderately competitive colleges. Also, consider a college's racial composition, extra-curricular opportunities, geographic location, availability of appropriate community and cultural activities, safety, general support services for minority students, tuition and fees, average financial aid / scholarship the school might provide.

As you are thinking about what you are looking for in a college, attend college fairs and see which schools fit your preferences. In addition, your local public library has college guides to help you obtain information. As you go through the listings look for application deadlines.

While in your library, be sure to investigate their scholarship books. Take the time to search through the books because a major scholarship could be waiting for you. Be sure to identify any scholarship application deadlines. In addition, there are situations were a more expensive college will provide more aid in scholarships and grants then a less expensive school. This can make the final cost of the more expensive school less then the cheaper school. Thus, consider applying to a few colleges that are more expensive.

In the spring of your junior year take the SAT and ACT standardized exams. Ask your guidance counselor for exact dates, locations, and obtain application materials. Never take the SAT or ACT exam without preparing! It is important that you make time to review material and practice answering questions in exam-like conditions. In preparation, you can consider taking an SAT/ACT preparation course such as offered in most major cities by Stanley Kaplan. Though the courses can be expensive, scholarships are available. You can also purchase review books from bookstores or go through such books found in your pubic library. Begin your review at least two or three months before the exam. It is very simple, the better you prepare the better you will do. Remember, consideration for admission into competitive schools is often determined by exam scores.

During the fall of your senior year, you will begin the process of applying to the colleges you have selected. It is important to take the time to complete the applications neatly. Some colleges require a written essay as a component of the application. Put time and effort into your essay. A well-written essay may be the deciding factor that gets you accepted into a competitive school. Lastly, fill out your applications early and do not wait till just before the deadline to submit your application. Doing so only leads to unnecessary anxiety and denial of admission to your school of choice.

Most applications have a financial aid component. As a result, it is important to be prepared. Most of the information is from tax returns filed by you and your parents. Become familiar with the "Free Application for Federal Student Aid forms" or FAFSA for short. This is the main set of documents required by most schools. Information about the FAFSA is found at www.fafsa.ed.gov of the Department of Education. In the event you have any questions call the college admission's office or ask your guidance counselor. No question is too dumb to ask.

During the spring of your senior year sit back and relax. Celebrate your acceptances. However, be sure to keep doing well in your classes. Most colleges require that your high school submit a final transcript and your acceptance is contingent upon maintained academic excellence.

Applying to College with a Pre-Medical Focus

As you consider your college selection, be sure to understand the college pre-medical education as described in the first two sections of chapter III. Briefly, a pre-medical student does not have to major in a science but can take advantage of a full liberal arts education. If you choose this, what else do you want to learn about? How about Black, Hispanic, or Native American studies; art, literature, history, dance, etc? As you have set upon medicine as your career choice this is going to be your best opportunity to learn and explore these other areas.

When you begin your college search, talk to students who have graduated from your high school with an interest in medicine and ask them about their pre-medical experience at the school they are attending. Once you have reduced your list of college choices, inquire about each school's pre-medical office. If there is one, give the pre-medical advisor a call and ask him or her some questions. Many schools have time set aside during the summer and fall for high school students to visit for a night or the weekend. If you have the time and money take advantage of these opportunities. Speak with the pre-medical students and advisor at the school. I guarantee that the time and effort spent going through this process will greatly reduce the possibility of frustration later on.

When considering college, there are a few things you need to think about. The first is how many minority students at that college or university continue to be pre-medical students after their first year and the number of minority students who apply to and/or are accepted to medical school each year from that college. If a college or university initially has a large number of pre-medical students and few of them end up applying to medical school and/or are accepted into medical school it means that they are falling between the cracks and there is a strong chance your fate may be the same.

Below are four reasons minority pre-medical students perform poorly while in college and do not make it to medical school:

1. The college lacks a pre-medical office. Pre-medical advisors are critical. They can help you select the right courses so you will be academically prepared to apply to medical school; can help find summer programs; can answer questions about the medical school application process; can write a letter of recommendation; and most importantly provide support to students who are going through the rigors of the pre-medial classes and the medical school application.

2. The school has a pre-medical office but the advisor is uncaring, uninterested, or even hostile toward minority students. If the advisor is not willing to support the student, then the student's ability to successfully navigate the pre-medical courses and then complete the application process becomes very difficult.

3. There are few minority pre-medical students at the college. When there are only a few minority students sitting in a pre-medical class that exceeds over a hundred students, it is very easy to feel isolated and alone. If a student is not ambitious, the environment may become overwhelming which can lead to a poor academic performance.

4. The minority pre-medical students do not work well together and there is a lack of commitment of the science faculty to ensuring the success of minority students. If the minority pre-medical students work together and support each other, there is a great chance you will do very well. In addition, if the science professors are willing to go out of their way to work with you on class work you probably will do well at that school.

BS – MD Duel Degree Program

Be aware of the universities and medical schools who sponsor this program. Often a student is accepted into the undergraduate college and the medical school at the same time (B.A. - M.D. or B.S. - M.D. dual degree program). There are some medical schools who have a special relationships with specific colleges and will accept a few select pre-medical students early.

Participation in this program has benefits. Some do not require their participants to take the Medical College Admissions Test (MCAT) or go through the regular medical school application process. Some programs allow their participants to take medical school classes after their 2nd or 3rd year in college allowing the student to save time and money.

Often, admission is very competitive. However, do not hesitate to submit an application. You have nothing to lose. Participation in a dual degree program requires attendance at one school from six to eight years. For some, this is too much time to be at one school or location. The curriculum is often very structured and participants do not have the opportunity to explore the liberal arts education.

To search schools that participate visit: http://services.aamc.org/currdir/section3/degree2.cfm

Do I have what it takes to be Successful?

As a high school student, the future may be a bit confusing and intimidating. Medicine is nice but is there some hesitation in your mind to pursuing such a lofty goal? You are not the first to feel this way. Take a few minutes and read the ten biographical essays located in the appendix. Pre-medical students come from a variety of backgrounds and experiences. Yet, many participated in a medical experience, were student leaders, did well in their classes, and realized that fulfilling the dream of becoming a physician required hard work, commitment, and perseverance. Does this describe you?

You may receive advice from a counselor or teacher to choose an alternative less demanding health career field. Take this advice seriously but ask many questions. If you have done the research, obtained exposure to medicine, and your grades are strong or steadily improving, then remain steadfast. Enter college with the determination to raise your "game" to a higher level.

Realistically though, not all high school graduates are ready for college. Additional time is required to mature. Consider training as a Certified Nursing Assistant (CNA), Medical Assistant (MA), or Licensed Practical Nurse (LPN). Get your foot in the health care door. When you are ready, enter college focused and determined. Entering college with the training of an MA, LPN, or CNA can be a financially savvy decision. No matter where you attend college, there is likely going to be a medical facility where you can work. With the flexible hours many facilities provide, you might be able to work yourself through the college of your choice and graduate with little or no debt.

Becoming a Physician

Below is a list of the most successful colleges at producing minority medical school applicants based upon data from the AAMC: Minorities in Medical Education: Facts & Figures 2005.

Top 10 Colleges Producing African American Medical School Applicants for the year 2004

1. Xavier University
2. Howard University
3. Spelman College
4. Hampton University
5. Cornell University
6. Florida A&M University, Tallahassee
7. University of Florida, Gainesville
8. University of Michigan, Ann Arbor
9. Duke University
10. University of California, Los Angeles

Top 10 Colleges Producing Native American Medical School Applicants for the year 2004

1. University of Oklahoma, Norman
2. University of Arizona, Tucson
3. University of New Mexico, Albuquerque
4. Stanford University
5. Oklahoma State University, Stillwater
6. University of North Carolina, Pembroke
7. University of California, Los Angeles
8. University of Washington, Seattle
9. North Carolina State University, Raleigh
10. Northern Arizona University

Top 10 Colleges Producing Mexican American Medical School Applicants for the year 2004

1. University of California, Los Angeles
2. Stanford University
3. University of Arizona, Tucson
4. University of New Mexico, Albuquerque
5. University of Texas at Austin
6. University of California, San Diego
7. University of Notre Dame
8. University of California, Davis
9. University of Southern California
10. University of California, Santa Barbara

Top 10 Mainland Colleges Producing Puerto Rican Medical School Applicants for the year 2004

1. University of Florida, Gainsville
2. Columbia University
3. Harvard University
4. University of Georgia, Athens
5. New York University
6. Rutgers University
7. Tufts University
8. University of Miami
9. University of South Florida
10. University of Michigan, Ann Arbor

Medical History Gazette

Vol 1, No 2• The First Source for Medical History •Columbia, S.C.

News Flash!

African Americans in Medicine:
The Journey Begins

When the soldiers raided West African villages to supply the trans-Atlantic trade with human cargo no one was left behind. As a result religious leaders, artists, musicians, farmers, village leaders, and medical specialists arrived upon the shores of the Americas. Like their white counterparts, some of the African medical specialists controlled disease through charms and conjuration. However, there were many that understood the medicinal value of a wide assortment of minerals, plants, and herb concoctions. Some even knew the method of inoculation designed to prevent the onset of disease and the practice of giving birth by caesarian section.[1]

On many southern plantations, slave holders found it necessary to provide some type of medical care to their slaves. Often, it was up to slave practitioners to take care of their fellow workers. In fact, it was not unusual for neighboring planters to borrow the services of Black doctors who were well known in the locality for their success as practitioners.

It is important to note that many of the Black practitioners were women. The women usually combined the duties of obstetrician with skill in preparing and dispensing medical herbs. Frequently these women were listed in plantation inventories as "Doctor".[2]

To some plantation owners and overseers, any type of knowledge among the slave population was a threat to the existing system. Any display of medical talent, skill, or knowledge would be met with extreme punishment. In almost all of the Southern colonies the slaves were prohibited from learning how to read and write. And, in the state of Tennessee the courts prohibited them from practicing medicine. Some slave owners realized that, "not all slaves were happy, sweet-tempered, and fun loving" and cases of poisoning White patients occurred in great numbers.[3]

In spite of the projected fear, there were individual healers and practitioners who continued to brave the potential punishment, even death itself, to bring medical aid and comfort to their people. As such these practitioners had to perform their duties in secret.

Some of the medicinal knowledge of the Negro was so important to the greater community that they were persuaded to reveal their secrets. In South Carolina, **Caesar** was known for his cure for poison. On February 12, 1751, the

> The first professionally educated African American physician, James McCune Smith, earn his medical degree in 1837.

See **Journey** Next Page

State legislature ordered his prescription to be published for the benefit of the public. It was printed in the South Carolina Gazette of Charleston and the demand for this edition exceeded the supply. Caesar is known to have escaped to Massachusetts and in 1772 he wrote an article in the Massachusetts Gazette about the symptoms and treatment for poison.

Onesimus is known for having described a procedure in which he was given a weakened dose of smallpox which prevented him from getting the disease. Despite an initial unpopular response, it was this practice of inoculation that was adopted.

Of the free Black men and women of the North, **Lucas Santomee Peters**, is recognized as the first known African trained physician in the colonies. He studied medicine in Holland. He then returned to America and in 1667 received a grant of land in recognition of his services to the people residing in New Amsterdam (now known as New York).[4,5,6]

Despite the success of a few Black Americans living in the North, few rights or opportunities were provided. Thus, many of the early well known "doctors" like **James Still**, **William Wells Brown**, and **David Ruggles** were self-taught healers. David Ruggles had developed such a successful hydrotherapy treatment and facility that even William Lloyd Garrison, a pioneering white abolitionist, sought him out.

Though it did not happen often, some free Blacks living in the north had the opportunity to be apprentice educated physicians which was the custom method of training. Some of the apprenticed trained physicians include Drs. **John Rock** and **Martin R. Delany**.

Even less numerous than the apprenticed trained practitioners were professionally educated physicians. The first professionally educated African American physician, **James McCune Smith**, had to attend the University of Glasgow, Scotland, to earn his medical degree in 1837.

It was not until 1847 that the first African American, **David J. Peck**, graduated from an American medical school, Rush Medical College in Chicago. It took another seventeen years for the first African American woman to graduate from an American medical school, **Rebecca Lee Crumpler** in 1864. (It is interesting to note that at this time a medical education consisted of two years of lecture and training.)

Though all the physicians were dedicated to their medical practices, few were able to separate their dedication to healing the body from healing the social system. These physicians were passionate advocates of Black equality and lent their medical talents and efforts to destroy the studiously cultivated myth of the racial inferiority of Black men and women. For some doctors such as Martin R. Delany and James McCune Smith, the drive to crush slavery and the perception of Black inferiority was so great they all but gave up practicing medicine. Instead, Drs. Delany and Smith used their precious time and knowledge to travel and educate audiences about the real truth.

Chapter III

Pre-Medical Planning: The College Years

It is never to early to plan for medical school. Due to extreme competition, only 49.4% of the 35,735 applicants were accepted in 2004 to allopathic medical schools.[1] The more you plan your undergraduate career and understand the application process, the better your chances of being accepted by the medical school of your choice.

The five major areas you need to think about in planning your pre-medical career include: 1. The pre-medical program, 2. College major, 3. Extracurricular activities, 4. Summer activities, and 5. Enhancing your studying technique.

When entering college one of the most important decisions you will have to make is selecting an undergraduate major. The decision becomes even more complicated when you begin to think about trying to include the academic requirements for medical school. Therefore, the first item of importance on your agenda is to understand the pre-medical program.

The Pre-Medical Program

The medical profession is searching for students with scientific capabilities. Pre-medical student's are challenged to successfully complete a broad spectrum of science and English courses. These courses are as follows:

Subject	Semester or Equivalent	Lab
General Biology	2	Yes
Inorganic Chemistry	2	Yes
Organic Chemistry	2	Yes
Physics	2	Yes
English	2	No
Mathematics*	2	No
(*Achieve a level up to elementary calculus)		

A thorough understanding of the basic concepts and theories relating to electricity, current, resistance, diffusion, gas laws, ohm's law, acids, bases, buffers, electrolytes, pH, osmolality, chemical structures, titration, and many other topics are expected. All pre-medical students should be able to

17

effectively acquire, synthesize, apply, and communicate this information.

It is important to understand that the subjects/courses listed above are the only ones that are required for admission into medical school. In retrospect, I have found that taking physiology and genetics for the general biology requirements can be extremely beneficial in helping ease the academic transition into medical school. At least a quarter of the general medical school curriculum is based upon information presented in these two subjects. Though not required, exposure to biochemistry can also be extremely helpful. Other optional courses that provide some insight into the science of medicine include anatomy, histology, cell biology, embryology, and microbiology.

In addition to these particular courses, one should have a basic understanding and be comfortable using computers. In almost every medical school program, computers are integrated into the curriculum. In the future, virtually every aspect of medical care will utilize computers in some capacity. Take the time to learn how to use the computers to which you have access.

The six pre-medical subject areas were selected because successful completion of these courses will provide a student with a strong foundation from which they can understand material presented in medical school. Many times throughout my pre-medical career, I questioned whether I would ever use the scientific concepts taught in my pre-medical courses. In retrospect, the answer is mostly yes. I say 'mostly' because there is a chance you will not see or use some of the material again. However, that chance is based upon the medical specialty you decide to enter. Many medical students go into medical school with one specialty in mind and end up leaving medical school with an area of interest that is completely different. Completion of these subject areas prepares you with the foundation to enter whatever field you choose. Having a broad base of knowledge increases your ability to deepen your understanding of all subjects as new knowledge is added through your experience.

College Major

As you can see from the pre-medical program requirements, one does not have to major in biology, chemistry, physics, or any other science in order to be admitted into medical school. Therefore, choosing a science major solely because you think it will enhance your chances of getting into medical school is not in your best interest—especially if you do not have a strong interest in any particular field of science.

If you decide that you want to major in the humanities or social sciences, plan your academic schedule during your first and second year so that your pre-medical courses, the courses for your major, and the core requirements, do not conflict with each other. The time and effort spent planning your academic career will reduce the headache and frustration you may face later on.

The extra work you put toward planning your academic career so you can have a non-science major will be rewarded by your gain in knowledge and expertise in an area few of your pre-medical school peers will have. Note that as the movement toward primary care medicine continues, there is added interest in producing doctors who not only have a strong scientific background but also a strong humanities, social science, or liberal arts background from which they will be able to better understand their patients and be able to treat them as people. Additionally, the college years are the only time you will have the opportunity to study about your history, culture, and the people who came before you. Do not deny yourself this opportunity to gain a deep sense of pride along with the academics.

Medical schools are most concerned with the overall quality and scope of your undergraduate work. If you are a science major, studies in the humanities and the social and behavioral sciences are recommended. In addition, I also recommend that you develop effective writing and speaking skills. Honors courses and independent study or research is encouraged. They allow you to obtain a unique scholarly experience which will facilitate a lifelong habit of self-education.

Profile of 2004 Applicants to Medical School

Undergraduate Major	Applicants
Biological Sciences	57.7%
Physical Sciences	12.3%
Social Sciences	11.8%
Humanities	4.0%
Math/Statistics	0.9%
Health Sciences	3.4%
Other*	9.8%

*Includes: dual major's non-science and science/non-science, general science, general studies, honors program, and interdisciplinary studies.

It is very important that you speak with your pre-medical advisor, your advisor in your major, and upper class pre-medical students as soon as possible. They all should know the academic program very well. As a result, they can help you sort out the scheduling problems you will face. During your first year, if possible, you should map out your pre-medical career. Decide when you are going to take your biology, chemistry, physics, math, and English courses. If you plan well, you will be able to distribute your workload. This will prevent you from having to take an extremely heavy course load at any one time. If you plan well, there will be room for schedule changes in the future.

Not all chemistry, biology, math, or physics courses are the same. They tend to be unique because different professors teach them. Be sure to ask your fellow pre-medical students which professors are the most dedicated to working with students.

Many colleges provide their students with flexible grading options such as taking a class for either a grade or pass-fail. If this option is available to you, take all of your pre-medical courses for a letter grade. This allows medical school admissions committees the opportunity to evaluate your performance at a level that is comparable with other applicants. When you are in college, know how your academic performance will be presented on your transcript. Some colleges will not include courses you withdrew from or failed, while others will. If your transcript includes courses you withdrew from, be aware that frequent withdrawals do not sit favorably with medical school admissions committees. To prevent this from occurring, plan your academic schedule so it is not so difficult that you will have to withdraw from a course.

There is much concern among pre-medical students about grades, the grade point average, and admission to medical school. According to the Association of American Medical Colleges, the average minority student accepted into an allopathic medical school in 2002 had a 3.30 average in their pre-medical courses and a 3.57 average in their other courses.[3] The combined grade point average is about 3.43. It is important to use these averages only as a guide for your academic performance; do not set your academic goal just to meet the average. It is important to remember that these and other numbers presented are just averages. Thus, there are some applicants who had higher GPA's but were not accepted into medical school and some who had lower GPA's and were accepted into medical school.

The nature of your overall record is important - students who improve their performance after a poor start are looked upon more favorably than those whose records decline in the later more demanding courses. Students taking demanding sequences of science and non-science courses are looked upon more favorably than those who take large numbers of introductory courses in a variety of subjects or who elect "safe - sure A" courses.[4]

Extracurricular Activities

Medical schools look for some indication that an applicant has seriously investigated the medical profession. They check to ensure the student is aware that medicine is a very demanding and stressful profession. Involvement in pre-medical societies and taking the time to work or volunteer in a hospital, clinic, or other health care setting will prove to be enriching, exciting, and give you a flavor of what you will see and experience in the future.

Working within other student organizations, on sports teams, dance troupes, etc. can provide you with valuable leadership and organizational skills, as well as fun and excitement to break up the monotony of going to class everyday. Such experiences can only enhance your medical school application. They also give you the chance to learn how to interact with a variety of people, which is what you will be doing as a health care professional.

Keep in mind that whatever you do, your academic program must come first. If you become over committed and do poorly, medical schools will view this as an indication that you are unable to effectively budget and organize your time. Having the ability to organize ones time is crucial in determining ones success as a medical student and later on as a physician. In addition, admissions committees are not impressed with extensive lists of extracurricular activities but rather like to see a short list of activities in which you were able to make a meaningful and substantial contribution of time and energy.

Summer Activities

An often-unrecognized component of enhancing an application for medical school occurs during the summer months. Many economically endowed students are able to use this time to volunteer in hospitals and gain medical experience. However, there are many who do not have the opportunity to volunteer because of a need to earn money for the next school year. With this in mind, it is important to know that many summer programs provide their participants with enough economic assistance to cover living expenses while also providing stipends upon completion of the program. In addition, some programs provide travel expenses. So, if you live on the east coast and the program is on the west coast, your flight will be paid for.

Summer programs provide you with: a way to earn some money during the summer, a chance to travel to different parts of the country, a chance to network among fellow pre-medical students, a chance to meet some outstanding physicians of color, give you an opportunity to have your name included on a published research paper, and enhance your medical school application. Such programs also provide you with individuals who can write strong medical school recommendations. Having interacted with them more than you may have with any teacher at your school, they will be able to give the medical school a first-hand account of your capabilities. Of course, it's up to you to provide the glowing examples of these capabilities for them to write about!

Having research experience and/or some type of medical experience will give a medical school admissions committee a clear indication that you are serious about your medical ambitions. From such experiences you will also be better prepared to decide what field of medicine you want to do, or at least what you don't want to do.

Finally, summer programs provide a great opportunity to check out a medical school in which you might be interested. If a particular school of your interest offers a summer program to which you are accepted, obviously your participation will allow you to gain first-hand information about that school essentially free of charge.

Many medical schools sponsor summer programs specifically for minority pre-medical students. Such programs range from doing research, to public health, to enhancing your scientific background, and are located throughout the country. Call up any local or distant medical school and ask for their admissions office or office of Minority affairs / programs. Also, note that some hospitals sponsor summer opportunities for undergraduate students.

A great source of information is the book: "Minority Student Opportunities In United States Medical Schools" by the Association of American Medical Colleges. This book is updated biennially and may be purchased for $12.00 via the AAMC at Department 66, Washington, DC 20055 or by calling (202) 828-0416. Also look at www.aamc.org (section on publications and then browse a topic applicants). When considering Osteopathy, The American Association of Colleges of Osteopathic Medicine (AACOM) offers an extensive list of publications and resources. You can visit their web site at: http://www.aacom.org/home-applicants/index.html. It takes some time and effort to seek out these great summer programs but your persistence will be rewarded. Also, do not forget to stop by your pre-medical office for posted opportunities and talk to junior and senior pre-medical students to find out about programs they might have been involved in. Through these sources, you will learn about some great opportunities that are available to you.

Enhancing Your Studying Techniques

In addition to the four areas already outlined, you should begin to think about your study habits; once medical school begins you do not want to have to reorganize the way you study. The major problem student's face in medical school is the volume of material they are required to learn. The sheer volume of material that must be mastered in medical school far exceeds any undergraduate demands. This is made even more difficult because medical students are expected to not only know the general concepts and principles but also facts and detail. Due to the volume of material and the detail, medical students often face major time constraints. If a medical student approaches his or her studies in an inefficient and highly unproductive manner, then the challenge may seem impossible.

Since I began my studies at medical school, I noticed that a common philosophy existed among my peers. My peers did not study to pass a test or receive a letter grade, but rather studied to learn and understand the material. (Cramming before an exam will allow a student to use their short term recall and pass an exam. However, this does not promote long term knowledge retention and will not provide a solid foundation for future courses.) My peers and I realized that people's lives are going to be at stake. And, we were not going to allow someone's life to slip through our fingers because we did not know the basic material.

I also noticed that my peers are active learners. An active learner is someone who is prepared to learn. An active learner attends class activities and pays attention. An active learner is someone who doesn't hesitate to ask questions before, during, or after class. An active learner is someone who engages his/her instructor in discussion about the concepts until they have complete understanding. An active learner makes sure that the education he or she receives is worth the money and the time being spent.

Over the course of your undergraduate career, you should ask yourself if you are an active learner. Medical school admissions committees look for active learners because they understand that when medical school ends the educational process continues. Every day of every month of every year is another school day. New techniques, drugs, and information are generated daily. It is the physician's responsibility to keep up with the new information. The patients expect you to know the current information so they can receive the best possible care. One of the qualities which allow a physician to do this is their being an active learner.

During your college years you should think about how you study and what methods you can pick up to become an active learner. Do not be afraid to ask your peers about their study methods; a component of their study program may be just the thing you need to maximize your own study time.

However, do not be alarmed or feel left out if what works best for you is not the standard procedure. If you work on improving your study skills early in your educational career you will find that later on you will be able to learn more material in a shorter amount of time, which will give you more time to participate in other activities.

A Sample Study Program

After I entered medical school, a study program was introduced to me by Marcia Z. Wile, Ph.D. who was the Director of Curricular Evaluation at Case Western Reserve University School of Medicine, Having heard how successful her study program had been for other medical students, I chose to try it out myself. This was s great decision. The program dramatically improved the quality of my studying. I only wish the study program had been introduced to me early in my educational career. Below is a description of the study program.

Preparing to Take a Course

Before you step into the classroom, for the first day of class, you should be able to answer the following three questions:
1. What are my objectives for taking this course?

2. How does this course fit into my long term goal of getting into medical
    school and becoming a successful doctor?
3. How will this course enhance my body of knowledge and awareness?

Answering these three questions will allow you to develop a sense of purpose for the course you are about to attend.

As you journey through your pre-medical career, it may be very difficult to answer these three questions as you evaluate your pre-medical courses. If you encounter this obstacle, seek your advisor and bring up this issue. After the discussion, you should be able to answer the three questions for each of the courses. Having an understanding of the importance of the pre-medical courses and their purpose toward helping you achieve your goal, you will find that your motivation to study and maintain academic excellence in each of the courses will parallel your motivation and drive to get into medical school and becoming a physician with a solid scientific background.

Once you have determined your objectives for the course, the next step is to understand how the material will be organized and presented. When the course begins, the instructor should provide each student with a course outline. The course outline generally contains a list of all the topics that will be covered, when the topics will be presented, corresponding readings, and a list of laboratories and small group sessions. Take a few minutes to examine the list. Develop an understanding of the direction of the course by focusing on the main topics presented. In addition, develop an understanding of how each classroom activity will help you understand the topics presented.

Establishing a Framework for Learning

A good study program provides a student with the ability to maximize their college education. There are three steps to successfully carry this out: 1. Preparation 2. Attendance 3. Review.

1. Preparation:

Before attending each class, small group session, and laboratory, determine what topics will be discussed and, if possible, what key concepts you are expected to learn. Skim all reading material that correlates with the classroom activity. If the instructor does not point out key concepts for you to learn for lecture material, many textbooks include a list of review questions at the end of each chapter. If there are review questions, quickly read over them to determine what the author believes are the key pieces of information for the topic presented. As you skim the chapter look for the answers to the questions. In addition, be sure to look at the charts, graphs, and pictures. If the chapter has highlighted words be sure to look up those that are unfamiliar.

This preliminary work does not have to be time intensive; initially it may take 30 to 45 minutes. As your skills improve 15 to 30 minutes is all it takes. Extensive time is not needed because the goal of pre-class preparation is only to gain familiarity with the topic.

After this review, you will be able to 1.) determine your familiarity with the topic, 2.) know how the topic relates to material previously covered, and 3.) know how difficult the material will be for you to master. Lastly, this review of the reading material will give you a chance to assess how well it is written. If the material is poorly written, you will be alerted to pay close attention to the classroom lecture and discussion. When you attend class with some familiarity of the topic(s), you will be able to recognize the words and concepts as they are presented. Thus, you can be an active learner from the start.

2. Attendance:

Attending class, small group, and laboratory sessions is very important to this study program. When many students consider the learning process, the first thought that often comes to mind is going to the library to sift through class notes, and reading textbooks. Rarely do students consider their class activities as real knowledge gaining experiences. As a result, students often passively participate in class activities. In actuality, class activities should be an integral component of the educational experience. This is the time you should begin to acquire a firm foundation of the material. When you are able to incorporate class activities into the knowledge-gaining process, you will have more free time.

To further the knowledge-gaining process, the educational system is set up so that during each educational activity (class, small group, laboratory session, etc.) there is usually an individual who has 'content expertise'. This individual can be the professor or a graduate student / teaching assistant. This person can enhance your knowledge-gaining process by being able to re-explain concepts you do not understand and go in depth on late breaking material. Textbooks only explain concepts in one way, do not answer questions when they arise, and often are out of date a few years after they are published.

An important goal while participating in class activities is to walk out of the activity with a 'take home message' that will enhance recall of important concepts presented. Often students get into the habit of trying to copy down everything the professor says or writes on the board. When some students try to do this the notes become illegible due to poor hand writing or can be considered as half-notes because the instructor erased the material before it could be all copied down. In addition, students who try to copy everything down fail to listen to the content being presented. Thus, a student may be actively listening but not actively learning and understanding the material.

If you experience these problems, the pre-class review is very important. Having reviewed your pre-class readings you already know what definitions, charts, graphs, equations, molecular structures, etc will be presented. When the instructor writes something down you will recognize that it is already written down for you in your class readings and thus there is no need to copy it down. Just make a note that the structure, definition, equation, etc. was presented and you should be sure to look it over when you review after class.

3. Review:

After you attend your class, small group, or laboratory, review the material discussed that day. Go over your notes to refresh yourself on the main points and any particular concepts you need to look for when you review the assigned readings.

After you have finished reviewing your sources of information, it is time to put together a product of the days' learning. This product should integrate all the important concepts in your own words. It is important to record the information in your own words so that when you review this material for your mid-term exam, final exam, and even the MCAT exam, it will be presented in a format that you recognize because you wrote it.

The product that you put together should be in a format that fits your learning style. If you are an auditory person, use a voice recorder. If you are a visual person and love color, use colored pens and a specific color of paper. If you are artistic, documenting the material in a picture format may be your thing.

When you put together your 'product of learning', try to do as much of it from memory as possible. Like going to class, this should be considered a knowledge-gaining process and not end up as a copying exercise. Creating your product(s) of learning will help highlight the concepts you thought you understood but may still need a little more reviewing. You may also find that there are specific concepts you are still having a difficult time grasping. If this occurs, ask a fellow classmate to explain it to you, go see the professor during office hours, or go to the resource center the department has set up for students who have questions about their course material, if one is offered.

After two or three weeks into the course, you may notice that you have had to consult a number of outside resources because you are having difficulty understanding the main concepts. Such a situation may indicate that you need a tutor. Your college should have a tutoring system established. If your school does not, go to your instructor and have him or her pair you up with someone who can help you.

If you encounter difficulty in a class, it is important to seek help immediately. Do not be bashful about seeking help. Physicians do it all the time when they consult their peers with a patient's perplexing medical condition. If you sit on your problem, it may affect your ability to understand and learn future information. If you wait too long it may be difficult to recover.

Goals of the Study Program

There are three main goals to this study program. The first goal is concerned with the acquisition and retention of knowledge through a structured format. Before learning can begin, a student has to be prepared to learn. Preparation for class, small group, and a laboratory session will position a student to be an active participant in their own learning. The products of learning will reinforce concepts presented earlier and put the information in a format that will facilitate quick and easy recall at a later date. This framework will facilitate the development of a strong liberal arts education with a foundation in the math and sciences. From this foundation you will be able to understand concepts presented later in your educational career.

The second goal of the study program is to stay current and study efficiently. There is a large variety of activities to get involved in while in college. As a result, many students become over committed and do not stay current with their studies. Instead, they try and learn the material in a few short days before the exam. Students may do well on the exam but their ability to recall material a couple months after the exam will be very low.

Even if you adopt this study schedule or a modified version of it, you will experience times when you are unable to stay completely current. What you should do is put the material presented in past lectures which you have not gone over to the side and continue to prepare for present class activities; attend the class activities and review after class as though you were up to date. That way you continue to learn new material as effectively as possible. To catch up on old material, you will have to include additional study time to your schedule. By doing this you will only miss a little bit of information and will not be behind a lecture or two for the whole semester or until the next exam.

To study efficiently you need a proper preparatory and review environment. Find a quiet place with as few distractions as possible; in front of the television will not do. If you need music or background noise make sure that it does not prevent you from focusing on your studies.

The third goal of this study program is to enjoy your educational experience. Studying is important, but do not forget to always devote some time for yourself; do something that makes you happy such as working out, reading a book, being with friends. Also, remember that if your body is going to stay healthy it needs good food and sleep! To maintain a good balance between your educational experience and personal well-being, establish priorities and keep to them. If you find that 24 hours in a day are not enough, a change is needed. Work on developing good time management skills and establish a schedule for yourself.

Conclusion

In the beginning, this study program may seem very time consuming. However, you will find that the time needed to prepare for class will be less as you fine-tune your skills. In addition, the time spent after class reviewing will be reduced as you develop your ability to learn material while attending class activities. Thus, in the end, this study program will end up saving you time, will substantially increase your knowledge base, and will prepare you to be a physician with an excellent scientific background.

Becoming a Physician

Becoming a physician is a dream that requires taking many risks. Some will try to convince you the goal is unobtainable, too difficult, takes too much work, and will tell you with many words that you will never make it. As well, they will encourage you to play it safe and choose a profession that is easier to obtain and will produce instant riches. But, if you put your faith in God, pray, have patience, work hard, persevere, and keep your eye on the prize, you will achieve your dream of becoming a physician.

News Flash!

Medical History Gazette

Vol 1, No 3• The First Source for Medical History •Columbia, S.C.

Dr. James McCune Smith
Fights a War of Words Against Senator Calhoun

James McCune Smith was born in New York City in 1813. He received his primary education at the New African Free School, which had been established by the New York Manumission Society in 1787. Though extremely intelligent and bright, James was unable to matriculate to an American college. He moved to Scotland and in 1832 registered at the University of Glasgow. There, he earned a B.A. (1835) and M.A. degree (1836). Five years after entering the university, James received his Doctorate of Medicine becoming the first known Black American to receive a medical school degree.

> Dr. Smith defended his people against the racial inferiority myths that surfaced throughout the south.

Upon graduation, Dr. Smith returned to New York City and began to practice medicine. He built up a large practice and operated two pharmacies. In spite of his tremendous success at providing medical care, Dr. Smith spent less and less time practicing medicine and more and more time in the abolitionist movement.

Dr. Smith used his vast scientific knowledge and skill as a great writer and lecturer to defend his people against the racial inferiority myths that surfaced throughout the south and from the office of Senator John C. Calhoun, of South Carolina.

John C. Calhoun sought to support slavery by using statistics from the United States Census of 1840. According to the Census, "the first of its kind on the mentally ill, the rate of mental defectiveness among free Negroes was about eleven times higher than among Negro slaves."[1] It was concluded from the results that "The African is incapable of self-care and sinks into lunacy under the burden of freedom. It is a mercy to him to give him guardianship and protection from mental death."[2] Senator Calhoun also used anatomical idiosyncrasies such as brain size to conclude that "the Negro" mind is depressed and only functions instinctively.

In a memorial written to the Senate of the United States, Dr. Smith articulately showed that the Census numbers as they relate to the mental health of the "free Negroes" of the North were

See **Smith** next page

Smith: Continued from previous page

totally incorrect. He explained that many of the towns purported to have mentally ill "Negroes" had no "Negro" residents at all. He also went on to show that the number of mentally ill "Negroes" living in the North was proportionally equal to the number of white mentally ill.

Successfully winning the Census battle, Dr. Smith turned his attention to "Negro" inferiority based upon anatomy. Lecturing before a notable and prominent assembly of New Yorkers on "The Comparative Anatomy and Physiology of the Races." Dr. Smith was declared, by audience members, to have delivered the best argument assailing the "scientific" theory.

In addition to speaking throughout the North, Dr. Smith "brought fire to the pen". He wrote columns in the Colored American, a newspaper he edited, and the North Star, which was owned and operated by his friend Frederick Douglass. Due to his excellent writing abilities, Frederick Douglass asked Dr. Smith to write the introduction to his book, My Bondage and My Freedom.

Dr. James McCune Smith died in 1865 at the age of 52.

Black Physicians Refuse Push to Africa

In 1849, John Van Surly de Degrasse and Thomas J. White graduated from Bowdoin College with medical degrees. They were the second and third Black Americans to do so. They entered medical school under the auspices of the American Colonization Society. After graduation they were expected to travel and provide medical care to people living in Liberia, West Africa.

Upon finishing medical school, both refused to go. Instead, Dr. DeGrasse, who graduated with honors, traveled to Paris to study medicine, "under the teaching of the great lecturer and master of surgery", Alfred Armand Velpeau. He returned to the United States as a ship's surgeon on the S.S. Samuel Fox and established a medical practice in New York City. He then moved to Boston where he became so well known that on August 24, 1854, Dr. John V. Degrasse was admitted to the Massachusetts Medical Society. He became the first Black American to be admitted to a medical society.

Dr. John Sweat Rock Speaks out Against Slavery

He was born on October 13, 1825 of free parents in Salem, New Jersey. He was an avid reader and at age 19 served as a teacher in a one room school house. Two local physicians were impressed with John's intelligence and skill and he completed a two year medical apprenticeship under their guidance.

Despite numerous denials for admission to medical schools John was finally admitted to the American Medical College in Philadelphia, Pennsylvania. He earned his medical degree and then went on to attend to sick fugitive slaves passing through the city.

By the mid 1850's, Dr. Rock had moved to Massachusetts and was speaking out against slavery. From this he picked up a new profession: the law. On September 14, 1861 he received his license and could practice in all the state courts. He was so capable that on February 14, 1861 he was granted permission to argue cases before the United States Supreme court. He died on December 3, 1866.

Chapter IV

When Should I Apply to Medical School?

The majority of pre-medical students attend medical school straight from college. To accomplish this, the pre-medical courses are completed before the senior year. The Medical College Admissions Test (MCAT) is taken during the spring of the junior year. In the senior year, the medical school application and interviews are completed.

This is not the only available option. Consider the other options as described below and determine the best one for you. Just because one student decides to take one path does not mean that same path is right for you.

Studying Abroad and Taking Time Off

An important aspect of many college careers is studying abroad. Many schools have programs for their students to study abroad during the junior year. If you plan your pre-medical education, there is no reason why you cannot take advantage of this exciting opportunity. Choosing this option, though, will mean that you would have to take a year off between college and medical school. During the spring of your senior year you would take the MCAT exam. You would then to use the year off from school to apply for admission to medical school.

Even if you are not interested in traveling abroad during your junior year, you still may want to consider taking a year off before going to medical school. Often by the end of your senior year the last thing you want to think about is another school year and another year of classes. If you are interested in taking a year off you have two options.

The first option is to apply to medical school as though you were going to matriculate the year you graduate from college. However, arrange a deferment so you can begin medical school a year later. In considering this option, check with the medical schools you are interested in to see if they offer this option to their accepted students. The main benefit of the deferment option is that you will not have to complete the application and interview process during the year off and thus disrupt your activities. As well, the application process is much easier to complete while you are in college. If you need to take care of any unfinished business or problems arise, you can meet with your pre-medical advisor and take advantage of any support services your school may provide. Often it can be difficult and frustrating trying to complete important business over the phone and outside of the campus setting.

The second option you have is to begin the application process during your senior year as if you studied abroad during your junior year. During the spring you can take the MCAT exam and begin the medical school application process. The major benefit of this option is the additional flexibility it offers you in completing your pre-medical courses; you can use four years instead of three.

If you take a year off before medical school, have a plan of what you will do with your time. Some students use the time to travel while others find a job in a research lab. Whatever the decision, make the time meaningful. If you have undergraduate loans, it is important to be aware that after graduation you will have a short grace period, typically six months, before you are expected to begin making loan payments. However, once you begin medical school, your loans payments can go into deferment until you finish medical school and residency.

One question that often comes up when considering time off between college and medical school is retention of knowledge. The best way to approach this is to examine how you studied for your pre-medical courses. If you typically "crammed" the night before an exam, your retention of knowledge is going to be minimal and there is some reason for concern. However, if you studied to understand the concepts and did not cram the night before, you may not have much of a problem. As well, some medical schools have pre-matriculation programs. In these programs, much of the basic material covered during the first year of medical school is reviewed. As you apply to medical schools, look back at your pre-medical career, your retention of knowledge, and MCAT scores. If they are average or a little below average you may want to consider going to a medical school which offers a pre-matriculation program.

Medicine as a Second Career

For some, the thought of medicine as a realistic career was far from reality during high school and college. Science and health classes may have been enjoyable but only as a passing hobby. However, following many years of work in some other profession the heart is left unfulfilled. It is realized that medicine is the true professional calling. Other individuals are intimately involved with a close relative or friend's illness. Such an experience introduced or reintroduced the medical profession. Of these people, the consensus was that medicine is the profession that best suits them. The only difference between these people and everyone else is that it took them longer to come to this conclusion.

If you see yourself in a similar situation, the pathway into the field of medicine is the same as if you were still in college. The pre-medical courses can be completed at a local college or university. The completion of all the courses generally takes a year and a half to two years. Then there is the application process and eventually medical school.

I include medicine as a second career when discussing when to apply to medical school, because the perfect time to apply to medical school is when you are ready. It is unrealistic to expect everyone to know what they want to do for the rest of their lives when they begin college or even finish college. Whatever your situation, never think that the medical profession is out of reach because you are a little older and have been out of college for a number of years. In fact, the percentage of medical students over the age of 28 comprises more than 12% of all first year students.[1]

As an older adult, you may be single/married with children. Though this can make the pre-medical and medical school processes a bit more difficult, it does not have to keep you from pursuing your interest in becoming a physician. If you are married, work out a plan with your spouse on how to incorporate the limited amount of time you will be able to devote to the family. Make sure that the burden and sacrifice is not placed on one person's shoulders and that the plan is suitable for everyone. Sacrifices will have to be made on the part of everyone; however, becoming a physician is an effort that is well worth the sacrifice. If you have children and are single, work out an arrangement with relatives and friends prior to matriculation so that you will be able to have the time you need to devote to your studies.

Trying to balance all the responsibilities of being a parent and/or spouse can be difficult; especially when one of the two is in medical school. When you begin applying to medical school it is important to make sure that the school you eventually choose gives you the maximum flexibility in maintaining your role as a parent. Important information to consider is the average age of the first year medical school class, the number of medical students with families and/or children, and the structure of the curriculum. Other important factors to consider include the availability of daycare and its proximity to the medical school, the community's public school system, the availability of family housing, and whether extra provisions in financial aid are provided to married students or students with children.

Do not worry,

Do not be anxious,

Pray, Trust, and Believe in God.

He will carry you through each and every situation.

News Flash!

Medical History Gazette

Vol 1, No 4• The First Source for Medical History •Columbia, S.C.

African American Women
Break the Color Barrier in Medicine

Often when we are exposed to the events of African American history we read about the achievements of Black men. Most people have heard the names Charles Drew and Daniel Hale Williams. But rarely have we heard or know the people behind the names Rebecca Lee Crumpler M.D., Rebecca J. Cole M.D., Matilda Arabella Evans M.D., Francis M. Kneeland M.D., and May Edward Chinn M.D. The following is a brief look at the lives and careers of some of America's most historic and dedicated female African American physicians.

The first Black woman to complete a medical course at an American University was **Sarah Mapps Douglass** (1806-1882). She attended the Ladies Institute of the Pennsylvania Medical University for three years and completed her studies in 1858. She became a founding member of the Philadelphia Female Anti-Slavery Society and was in charge of the girls' department of the Institute for Colored Youth in Philadelphia.

In March 1864, **Rebecca Lee Crumpler**[2] became the first African American women to obtain the Doctor of Medicine degree. Born in Richmond, Virginia, in 1833, Rebecca Lee was raised in Pennsylvania by her aunt. The aunt served as a "doctor" to her community. This influenced Rebecca to seek every opportunity to help others.

Between 1852 and 1860 Rebecca Lee worked as a nurse in Massachusetts. Upon the recommendation of her employers she was admitted to the New England Female Medical College in Boston. She successfully completed her studies and graduated with a medical degree in 1864.

Dr. Crumpler devoted her life's work to the study of diseases affecting women and children. In 1883 she published "A Book of Medical Discourses" which offered advice to women on how to provide medical care to their children and themselves.

Three years after Rebecca Lee Crumpler received her medical degree, 1867, **Rebecca J. Cole**[3] graduated from the New England Medical College becoming the second African American woman to receive a Doctor of Medicine degree.

Dr. Cole was born on March 16, 1846, in Philadelphia, Pennsylvania. She graduated

The first two African American women to receive a Doctor of Medicine degree graduated from the New England Medical College, Boston Massachusetts.

See **Color Barrier** next page

Color Barrier: Continued from previous page

from the Institute for Colored Youth whose purpose was to educate African Americans so they could become the teachers for the next generation of African American students. However, Reebecca had other plans and chose to uplift her people by pursuing a career in medicine. Devoted to social medicine, Dr. Cole practiced in Philadelphia and helped start the Woman's Directory which provided medical and legal assistance to women. Later, Dr. Cole moved to Washington D.C. and became superintendent of the Home for Destitute Colored Women and Children. Dr. Cole practiced medicine, for over 50 years, until her death in 1922, at the age of 76.

Susan McKinney Steward, born in 1847 in Brooklyn, New York, was admitted to the Women's Medical College of the New York Infirmary for Women and Children in 1867. Applicants had to demonstrate good English education, knowledge of elementary botany and chemistry, and to previously have been under the instruction of a physician. Susan was selected by her classmates and faculty as class valedictorian and graduated on March 23, 1870. She was the first Black woman in New York State and the third Black woman overall to receive a medical degree.

Dr. Steward was active in the King's County Homeopathic Medical Society. In her career she helped organize the Brooklyn Woman's Homeopathic Hospital and Dispensary, was a member of the medical staff of the New York Medical College and Hospital for Women, and worked as a college physician for Wilberforce University in Ohio. She died on March 7, 1918.

On May 13, 1872, in Aiken, South Carolina, **Matilda Arabella Evans** was born. Upon the urging of an instructor at the Schofield Industrial School, Matilda enrolled in Oberlin College in 1887. The administrators of the school were so impressed with Matilda's academic abilities, they awarded her a scholarship to cover her tuition. However, just three months before graduation, Matilda dropped out of college to pursue a career in medicine. She enrolled at the Woman's Medical College of Pennsylvania in 1893 and received her medical degree in 1897. Upon receiving her degree, Dr. Evans returned to South Carolina and became the first African American woman to practice in the state. Dr. Evans became a successful surgeon whose clientele grew so large that she turned her home into a small hospital.

In 1901, Dr. Evans gave up her lucrative and secure private practice and established the Taylor Lane Hospital and Training School in Columbia, South Carolina. Taylor Lane Hospital was the only institution that would serve the city's African American community which comprised 50% of the city. Besides providing deeply needed medical care to the Black community, the hospital proved to become an excellent training ground for Black doctors and nurses.

Over the course of her life, Dr. Evans not only was a great physician but also a great educator and humanitarian to her community. For her services Dr. Evans was awarded numerous awards and honors. In addition, she was elected president of the Palmetto State Medical Society and was elected Vice President of the National Medical Association.

Dr. Evans died on November 17, 1935, in Columbia, South Carolina, at the age of 63.

See **Color Barrier** next page

Color Barrier: Continued from previous page

Francis M. Kneeland, is one of the most pioneering Black women physicians to graduate from Meharry Medical College in Nashville, Tennessee. She graduated with honors in 1898, just five years after the first two Black women (Georgiana Patton, M.D. and Annie D. Gregg, M.D.) graduated from Meharry.

Dr. Kneeland set up her practice in Memphis, Tennessee, and became the first Black Woman to practice surgery and medicine in the state. As the only Black female doctor in the city, Dr. Kneeland was well known for her work in uplifting Black women. As a result, she was the favored physician of hundreds of women in the city as well as Black nursing students enrolled at the University of West Tennessee where she served as the head instructor.

Born in Washington, D.C., on September 17, 1900, **Lena Frances Edwards** was destined to achieve success.[6] She was valedictorian of her high school class and after college she went on to medical school. Lena received her medical degree in 1924 from Howard University College of Medicine and began her career in community practice. Early in Dr. Edwards' medical career she developed extensive skill at home deliveries which is how she began to establish herself as an expert in the field of obstetrics and gynecology. From 1931 to 1945, Dr. Edwards served as assistant gynecologist at the Margaret Hague Maternity Hospital in Jersey City, New Jersey. In part due to the work of Dr. Edwards, Hague Hospital had one of the leading Ob-Gyn clinics in the country.

In 1948, Dr. Edwards passed the oral examination of the American Board of Obstetrics and Gynecology making her one of the first African-American women certified in the specialty.

In 1959, Dr. Edwards went to Hereford, Texas and provided services for and subsidized the founding of Our Lady of Guadeloupe Maternity Clinic for Migrant Workers. It was because of her dedication to this effort that President Lyndon B. Johnson awarded her the Presidential Medal of Freedom.

Dr. Edwards received numerous other awards. In 1973 she was recognized and presented with an award for her efforts to introduce Pap smear screening to women with low incomes. The Medical alumni Association of the Howard University College of Medicine honored her as a "living legend" for her dedication to the school and for her contributions toward uplifting the health of the African American community. In addition, Dr. Edwards was awarded honorary doctorates from St. Peter's College in Jersey City and the University of Portland.

Dr. Edwards passed away on December 3, 1986, at the age of 86.

> In 1964, President Lyndon B. Johnson awarded Dr. Lena Frances Edwards, the Presidential Medal of Freedom, the highest civilian award for service.

Chapter V

Chapter V

Medical College Admissions Test (MCAT)

Like the SAT (Scholastic Aptitude Test) and the ACT, the MCAT is a test which is used to predict how well you will perform in medical school. Though the effectiveness of determining ones capabilities for future performance in medical school through this exam has been deeply debated, it is still used by medical school admissions committees to decide if a student will be granted an interview. Therefore, this exam must be taken seriously. Often we think that the quality and/or quantity of our extracurricular activities and a consistently good academic record will make up for a poor performance on the MCAT exam. This no longer is true. The competition for medical school is so tough that one has to be strong in all areas; extracurricular, academic, and MCAT.

The MCAT exam is offered two times during the year: spring (around April) and at the end of the summer (around August). All third year college students who want to enter medical school directly from college should take the exam in the spring. Students taking the exam in the spring will have their results before the medical school application season begins. Normally medical schools will not review an application until they have received the MCAT scores.

Registration for the MCAT exam opens approximately fifteen weeks before the exam is given. Early registration is recommended to obtain the test center of choice. The only way to register is online: www.aamc.org/mcat. The registration deadline for the spring exam is the middle of March and for the summer exam the middle of July. If you plan to apply to an allopathic medical school, your test scores will automatically be included with your AMCAS application (AMCAS described in chapter VI). However, if you are applying to a non-AMCAS school you can go online at http://services.aamc.org/mcatthx and specify the non-AMCAS school and application services to which your MCAT scores should be sent.

What is the MCAT?

The MCAT will assess your understanding of the material presented in your pre-medical science courses. It also assesses problem solving, critical thinking, and writing skills. The examination is divided into four sections. Two are taken in the morning and two in the afternoon with a break in between for lunch.

The four sections are as follows:

1. Verbal Reasoning - (85 Minutes) - Consists of 60 multiple-choice questions (9 passages with 6-10 questions/passage) on topics from the humanities, social sciences, and natural resources. These questions will be based on the information presented. Therefore, no prior knowledge of the material is needed.

2. Physical Science - (100 minutes) - Consists of 77 multiple-choice questions (10 problem sets with 5-10 questions/set and 15 problems) focused on physics and general chemistry. Typically, this section is composed of passages upon which the subsequent multiple-choice questions are based.

3. Writing Sample - (60 minutes) - Consists of two topics; 30 minutes allotted for each topic. The student is asked to develop a central theme, synthesize material, separate major from minor issues, propose alternative solutions, present a theme in a logical manner, and write in standard English.

4. Biological Sciences - (100 minutes) - Consists of 77 multiple-choice questions (10 problem sets with 5-10 questions/set and 15 problems) focused on biology and organic chemistry. Typically, this section is composed of problems upon which the subsequent multiple-choice questions are based.

Each section of the MCAT, except the writing sample, is given a score between 1 (lowest) and 15 (highest). The writing sample is given letters J (lowest) through T (highest).

Below is a profile of the scores for under-represented minority students in the 2004 applicant pool.

	MCAT Score
Verbal Reasoning	7.6
Physical Sciences	7.5
Biological Sciences	8.1
Writing (medial score)	O

The above scores can provide a guide of how well you need to perform on the exam to have a medical school seriously consider you for admission. However, always remember that these scores are averages, some students with lower scores are accepted, and some with higher scores are not accepted.

Preparing for the MCAT Exam

There are many resources available to prepare for the MCAT exam. No one source is best for everyone since preparatory needs vary from student to student. The two major strategies are to use an MCAT review book or utilize a commercial preparatory review course.

A Personal Review Program

The MCAT exam is based upon the pre-medical courses and your ability to write and comprehend the English language as used in exams. No other knowledge is required. For the best result, begin preparing for the MCAT as soon as you begin college. Take your pre-medical math, science, and English courses seriously.

Students who do well in their pre-medical courses are often in the position to tutor other students. Tutoring other students in the pre-medical courses is an excellent way to review and master material. Tutoring is a valuable experience because the student will often force the tutor to look at the scientific concepts from various perspectives. Having a multi-dimensional understanding of the pre-medical material will prove to be a tremendous asset when taking the MCAT exam. Tutoring also has its financial rewards. Many schools will pay tutors for their time and effort.

If you have learned the main concepts in your pre-medical courses as described above, use of a self-instruction MCAT review book may be all you need. There are many review books available. Stop by your local bookstore or go "on-line" at amazon.com and review the books available. The Association of American Medical Colleges (AAMC) offers resources that complement many of the review books. The AAMC has made multiple full-length practice exams for the MCAT available to pre-medical students. The exams are available in print or on the web. These exams are critical because not only do they provide real questions but also explanations for the correct answers. One component of a good preparatory strategy is to practice taking multiple-choice questions under strict exam-like conditions. When you take the exam, you may know the material but the questions could mislead you if you are not familiar with the wording and/or presentation. Practice with these exams will prevent this from occurring. You can find the AAMC exams at: aamc.org/publications/start.htm and under "browse a topic" click on applicants. These practice exams cost about $40.00 each. If you visit www.e-mcat.com a free exam can also be found.

Finally, in considering a self-review course you should think about your ability to maintain a study schedule and your motivation. If you are disciplined, can establish and maintain a review schedule, and have the ability to motivate yourself to study even when the exam is one or two months away you will have no problem carrying out this course of study.

A Commercial Preparatory Review Program

A preparatory review course such as that presented by Stanley Kaplan (www.kaptest.com) or Princeton Review Inc. (www.princetonreview.com) has been used by many students. The main advantage of these review programs is that they are very structured. The Kaplan review course is about eight weeks. The curriculum consists of a combination of lectures, home study notes, and practice exams. PhD candidate students or college graduates who excelled in any one of the pre-medical fields generally teach the lectures. The lectures are often held at the "education center". Home study notes are provided to supplement the lectures. Some participants describe these notes as the most beneficial aspect of the review program. The practice exams consist of tapes and written exams. The tapes have a volume of questions in each of the subject areas. The tapes are available for student use anytime the center is open. When the review program begins, students take an exam to help evaluate which areas are their weakest. Throughout the review course written exams are given. Participants can use the exams to assess their proficiency in each of the MCAT exam segments.

Choosing to take a preparatory course is often a difficult decision. Some students who are not self-motivated appreciate the course because it forces them to establish a review program and maintain it. Other students have not liked the review course because it did not meet expectations based on the course's expense. The best way to decide if you need this type of review is to talk with students who have taken the course and consider your ability to complete a self-review course. If you have a choice between courses be sure you compare them thoroughly. Some courses may have a strong pre-medical course review but fall short in terms of providing tests that would challenge a student at a level of difficulty comparable to the MCAT. For the location of testing centers in your area, please visit the corresponding web pages.

MCAT Summer Programs

If you do enough research, an additional alternative may be available to you. Some medical schools sponsor MCAT review summer programs for minority students. Such programs can be especially helpful because they provide individual attention and a longer time span to review the material. Some programs may have enough funding to provide you with a stipend so that you would not have to miss earning a summer income. The best place to begin searching for such programs is to contact your pre-medical office.

Strategies for Taking Multiple Choice Exams Like the MCAT

Before entering the exam center to take the Medical College Admissions Test, you should have established a strategy that will enable you to achieve the best score possible. As I explained in the introduction of this chapter, medical schools admissions committee's use the MCAT to assess your ability to successfully pass standardized multiple-choice exams. During medical school, a student is required to pass two standardized multiple-choice exams, called the United States Medical Licensing Exam (USMLE) part I and II, before they can graduate.

Below are some important points to remember as you establish a strategy for taking the Medical College Admissions Test.

1. Knowledge is the Key to Success:

There is nothing in the world that can get you through the exam more then having a broad knowledge base. As you go through your pre-medical courses obtain as much knowledge as you can. As difficult as the material may seem don't let any page remain unturned.

2. Question Familiarity:

Be sure that you are familiar with the different types of questions that will appear on the exam before you take the real exam. As you review the questions, look for key words such as "true", "false", "except", and "least". If you have difficulty with one type of question be sure to spend extra time practicing that type of question.

3. Reading Questions:

Most questions are written in a very systematic fashion. Some information is presented, a question is asked based upon the information, and then a list of possible answers are presented. Normally we read each question in this format. This is problematic because as the text is read one does not know what information is important because the question / answer choices have not been presented. After reading the text and then the question and answers, we normally read the text again in order to identify important pieces of information. This is a time consuming process. Precious seconds can be saved by first reading the question and answers first. Then go back and read the text. As you read the text you should be able to circle the important words or phrases to help answer the question.

4. The "Best Answer":

As you answer each question, be sure to look at all the answers. Many questions are written with the seemingly obvious answer as the first or second choice. However, the question writers are often looking for the "best answer". This means that more than one answer could be correct, but one answer is more correct than another. The "best answer" can only be determined by reading all the choices.

5. Answer Each Question in Sequence:

Often people advise a test taker who does not know an answer to circle the question and then return to it after finishing the other questions. However, I suggest that if you are unsure of an answer that you make your best guess and move on. The first time you see a question you are more likely to answer it correctly using your initial thoughts. If you skip the question, you may run out of time and not have the opportunity to return to it. In addition, if you return to the question you will have to come up with your original thoughts that were circling in your mind. Also, by the time you come back to the question you probably will be very tired and will not be able to think about the question as clearly as when you saw it for the first time.

6. Guessing:

You will come across some questions that you have little or no knowledge about. As you contemplate the correct answer try to reduce the number of choices to as few as possible, make an educated guess, and then move on.

Even with questions that test information you have little knowledge about, it is possible to make an excellent educated guess. Answers that contain words such as "all", "only", "no", "never", or "always" generally suggest a false answer. Look for key words in the question that are repeated in the answer or contain a synonym of a key word found in the question and in one of the answers. Such words often target a correct answer. Lastly, questions that have a numerical answer often include false answers at each extreme high and low with the correct answer somewhere in the middle.

If you are not able to cross out any of the choices, answer the question using a pre-selected letter. For each question that falls in this category, continue to use the same pre-selected letter. Using the same letter will give you a greater chance of obtaining the right answer compared with randomly choosing a letter.

7. Changing Answers:

Once you have made your choice do not change any of your answers unless you know beyond all doubt that a different answer is correct. You have a greater chance of changing a correct answer to a wrong answer than the other way around.

8. Take Practice Exams:

Before you take the real exam be sure to take at least two practice exams in exam like conditions. This way you can establish a good intuitive pace that will allow you to complete all the questions but will not scare you into rushing so you finish the exam with too much time to spare. Practice exams can be a quality way to assess your strong and weak areas so you can make the most of your time spent reviewing.

Physical and Psychological Preparation for the Medical College Admissions Test

The Week before the Exam

Four or five days before you are scheduled to take the MCAT, you should begin to wind down your hectic preparatory schedule. If you have been staying up late, begin to go to bed earlier and get a good nights sleep.

Get some exercise during the weeks leading up to the exam. It is a great way to reduce some of the anxiety that naturally builds up in the body. In addition, on the day of the exam your body will be relaxed and able to get through a full day of inactivity that the exam day will bring.

Predetermine how much time you will need, on the exam day, to wake up, eat a good breakfast, and get to the exam station with time to spare; if you have to drive to the exam station give yourself a little extra time in case traffic is heavy. A few days before the exam, practice getting up at the hour you will get up on the exam day. This will allow your body some time to adjust if this means getting up at a new hour.

The Day Before the Exam

The day before the exam, try not to do any studying. Relax, see a movie, have fun with your friends, but do not do anything that will fatigue your mind.

In the evening, have a high carbohydrate dinner such as pasta. It is often a practice of long distance runners to eat pasta or some other high carbohydrate meal the night before a race because it provides the body with plenty of fuel the following day. Your mind will need all the energy it can have to get through the daylong MCAT exam. Also, never drink alcoholic beverages on the night before the exam. Doing so can disrupt your memory and affect your ability to recall important information. Before you go to bed, take the time to collect the items you will need for the exam:

- •Bring at least two or three #2 pencils (if needed).
- •A pillow can provide great comfort for the long day of sitting.
- •Some high-energy snacks will provide an extra boost.
- •A great packed lunch with all your favorites can hit the spot. They do not always place test centers close to restaurants.
- •Be sure that you have your admission ticket and any other materials you are required to present so you can enter the examination station.

The Day of the Exam

When you get up be sure to put on very comfortable clothes. As you take this exam, you are not graded on how you look. If you are unsure of the atmospheric conditions within the testing center, wear clothes that can be easily taken off or put on.

Be sure to eat a good breakfast. Breakfast will provide your body with the immediate energy to make it through the first morning segment of the exam without getting too fatigued and having your stomach growl.

During the exam breaks relax, have a snack, and unwind. However, do not join in a conversation with your peers or anyone else who choose to talk about questions and the answers they chose. If the discussion pertains to questions in which you chose answers that were slightly different from the consensus you may lose confidence in yourself and get flustered which can impact your performance on the rest of the exam. Lastly, relax. All you can do is your best and your best is what you will do.

Clinical physicians are private investigators.

They search into the heart, mind, soul, spirit,

and body to uncover each patient's ailment.

News Flash!

Medical History Gazette

Vol 1, No 5• The First Source for Medical History •Columbia, S.C.

Drs. Susan La Flesche Picotte & Lillie Rosa Minoka Hill Become America's First Native American Woman Physicians

Susan was born to Mary and Chief Joseph La Flesche on the Omaha Reservation in northeastern Nebraska in 1865. As a child, Susan is noted to have seen a sick Indian woman die after a local white doctor would not provide medical care. This experience inspired her to train as a physician so she could provide that care.

Until age 14, she went to school on the reservation. She then received some home schooling before she enrolled at the Elizabeth Institute for Young Ladies in New Jersey.

She returned home at age 17 and taught at the Quaker Mission School. At the school, she was encouraged to pursue her interest in medicine. She eventually enrolled at the Woman's Medical College of Pennsylvania in 1887. She graduated at the top of her class in just two years. Upon receipt of her medical degree, 1889, Dr. La Flesche became the First American Indian woman in the United States to receive a medical degree.

Dr. La Flesche spent one additional year in Philadelphia to complete an internship and then returned home. On the Omaha reservation, she provided healthcare at a government boarding school where she ran a busy medical practice.

In 1894, Dr. La Flesche married Henry Picotte and they moved to Bancroft, Nebraska where she worked in her own medical office, lobbied for the prohibition of alcohol on the reservation, and opened a hospital.

Dr. La Flesche died in 1915.

Lillie was born on the St. Regis Reservation in Northern New York State. Her mother is a Mohawk Indian and her father a Quaker physician from Philadelphia who worked on the reservation. Lillie's mother died at childbirth and she remained on the reservation till she began school.

At age five, she moved to Philadelphia where her father enrolled her in a Quaker school for girls. After high school, Lillie decided to be a nurse. However, her father encouraged her to work toward becoming a physician. She took this encouragement and in 1899 graduated from the Women's Medical College of Pennsylvania. She became the second American Indian woman to graduate from a medical school.

Dr. Minoka was married in 1905 to Charles Hill and they moved to an Indian

See **Dr. Minoka** next page

Dr. Minoka: Continued from previous page

Reservation in Oneida, Wisconsin. On the reservation, Dr. Minoka found that many of the people did not seek care from the current physician because he was white and did not understand their culture. She understood the needs of the people and slowly earned their trust. In 1917, the only licensed physician moved out and she was responsible for managing everything.

Never having officially obtained a medical license in Wisconsin, Dr. Minoka was limited in what she could do; but if it could be done, she did it. In 1934, Dr. Minoka sat for the state medical exam and upon passing, she received her medical license.

Dr. Minoka worked to prevent illness, promote sanitation, and delivered health and hope to the poor and underserved. Dr. Minoka died in 1952, but not before she had won numerous awards for her work.

Dr. Daniel Hale Williams Performs Historic Heart Surgery

On January 18, 1858, In Hollidaysburg, Pennsylvania, Daniel and Sarah Price Williams had their sixth child, Daniel Hale Williams. While Daniel was a small child, his family moved to Janesville, Wisconsin, where he grew into a bright enthusiastic young man.

Under the influence of a local physician, Daniel Williams was encouraged to study medicine. He began by serving as an apprentice to a doctor. A year later, he entered the Chicago Medical College (which later became Northwestern University). He received his M.D. degree in 1883.

Following graduation he entered practice as a surgeon for the South Side Dispensary. He also was a demonstrator of anatomy at Northwestern Medical school. At Northwestern, Dr. Williams became the first African American to serve on the faculty of an American medical school other than Howard and Meharry. By teaching at Northwestern, Dr. Williams acquired a thorough foundation in anatomy that enabled him to become an exemplary surgeon. In 1887, he was appointed a member of the Illinois State Board of Health and was reappointed in 1891.

Ten years out of medical school, Dr. Williams performed an historic operation. He carried out the first successful operation on the human heart; suturing of the pericardium. A newspaper wrote, "SEWED UP HIS HEART-Remarkable Surgical Operation on a Colored Man-At Provident Hospital-Dr. Williams Performs an Astonishing Feat-A Puncture in the vital Organ Exposed and Dressed with Success."

This same year, Dr. Williams left Chicago for Washington D.C. He was appointed by President Grover Cleveland to become Surgeon-in-Chief of Freedmen's Hospital. At the hospital, Dr. Williams reorganized the surgical department to such an impressive level that a previous Surgeon-in-Chief remarked that the "time had at last arrived when it is possible

See **Historic Surgery** next page

to penetrate the abdomen without fear". He also established a training school for nurses as well as bringing into existence a horse driven ambulance.

To reduce public fear of the "Negro" physician, Dr. Williams "threw open the doors of his operating room once a week to the public". He allowed anyone interested in watching a skilled surgical team, observe the operation performed in an amphitheater. Stiff opposition from some members of the medical community forced him to discontinue this practice.

In 1898, Dr. Williams left his post as Surgeon-in-Chief. From that time on he performed a variety of activities. In 1899 he began holding a surgical clinic at Meharry Medical College. Many at the school considered this to be the greatest annual educational event. From 1900 to 1906, Dr. Williams was an attending surgeon at the Cook County Hospital in Chicago and from 1912 until his death, he was associate attending surgeon at St. Luke's Hospital in Chicago. While he held each of these posts, Dr. Williams always traveled. He gave lectures and he annually traveled south spreading his knowledge.

Dr. Williams died in 1931 at the age of seventy-three (the patient whom Dr. Williams performed the historic operation on in 1893 is reported to have out lived him).

When Dr. Williams died, it is reported that he had developed a bitterness of spirit. His skill and ability was not seen by the dominant society to be an asset, but rather a threat. The color of his skin restrained continued advancement in the medical world proportional to his abilities; and Black America was not generally able to appreciate his contributions.

Though we have come a long way since Dr. Daniel Hale Williams' death, it seems as though the struggles and battles he had to fight are the same ones we are still fighting today.

Drs. Williams & Mossell Open
Nations First Black Run Hospitals

In the United States, the first major general hospital to open was Pennsylvania Hospital in 1751. This and other major hospitals often would not allow Black medical professionals to train and work in them. And, most provided meager care to Black patients who were isolated in an inferior wing of the hospital. Thus emerged the "Black Hospital".

On January 22, 1891, Provident Hospital located in Chicago Illinois opened its doors. Many believe that this was the first hospital in the United States to be fully operated by African Americans. Emma Reynolds was refused admission to multiple nurse training programs. Dr. Williams was sought out and agreed to work toward establishing Provident as a hospital where Black nurses could be trained and Black physicians could hospitalize their patients in the city of Chicago, Illinois.

On October 31, 1895 the Frederick Douglass memorial Hospital opened its doors at 1512 Lombard Street in South Philadelphia, Pennsylvania. The hospital opened with 65 beds and a staff of 20 nurses. Dr. Nathan Francis Mossell organized a team that raised $118,000 from among the Black community and a few benevolent white supporters.

Chapter VI

Successfully Choosing a Medical School

C hoosing a medical school is a difficult decision. Before making your selection, take the time to understand how the educational system works.

The Medical School Education

Medical schools are academic institutions that provide motivated students with the means by which to learn and understand how the body functions, what happens to the body when it becomes ill, and how to treat and manage these afflictions.

The Allopathic Medical Education

Allopathic medical schools traditionally divide their curriculum into two-year segments. The first two-year segment is devoted to study of the basic sciences which includes gross anatomy, cellular biology, embryology, molecular biology, biostatistics, histology, biochemistry, physiology, pathology, microbiology, neuroanatomy, immunology, genetics, epidemiology, pharmacology, physical diagnosis, behavioral science, and clinical laboratory procedures. These areas of medical science provide the student with the foundation to begin learning about clinical management of disease.

There are different approaches medical schools take in presenting their basic science curriculum. These approaches include the "traditional course based" approach, the "organ systems based" approach, and the "problem based" approach to learning. The traditional course based approach presents all information in a subject area, like gross anatomy, at one time. Often students take two or three courses at any one time. The organ systems approach presents all the basic science involving an organ system, such as the heart and blood vessels, in an interdisciplinary fashion. The problem-based approach requires students to work in small groups. Each group is presented with case studies to solve. In working through the case, each student learns the basic science related to the disease process presented.

In June, of the second year of medical school, all students take the United States Medical Licensing Exam (USMLE) Step I. This is the first of three standardized exams required for licensure to practice medicine in the United States. Additionally, passing this exam may determine whether a student will continue to the third year or will have to repeat some or all of the basic science medical education.

Between the first and second year, medical schools give their students an eight to ten week summer break. Medical students use this time in a variety of ways. Those who go to medical school directly from college, like to use this time to travel or just relax at home. Other students like to use this time to conduct research, shadow a physician, participate in a summer program, or take advantage of any other opportunity that may be available. This summer vacation tends to be a major event for medical students because it is the last time students will have a whole summer off during their medical education.

The third and fourth year of medical school, are devoted to clinical clerkships and electives. These give students the opportunity to work with patients in a hospital or in an outpatient clinic setting. Most clerkships consist of two to three month "rotations" through various departments, which normally include internal medicine, surgery, neurology, obstetrics/gynecology, pediatrics, psychiatry, and family community medicine. Some schools require students to complete a clerkship in radiology, dermatology, or ophthalmology as well. Each rotation helps students learn how to integrate the basic science of medicine with clinical care and medical decision making. The rotations give medical students a broad exposure to clinical medicine. This will help students make an informed decision on a career choice Electives provide the opportunity to explore areas of interest in detail. Some even allow a student to travel to medical facilities in other parts of the country or abroad. In the fourth year, medical students are required to take and pass the second part of the USMLE in order to receive their medical degree.

Early during the fourth year, students apply for placement in a residency program. Residency programs are similar to apprenticeships. It is here that the young doctor learns the fine details of his/her specialty under the supervision of a teacher. The length of time spent in training depends upon the type of specialty. Please see chapter XII "Careers in Medicine" for information on the medical specialties and length of residency training.

Allopathy (M.D.) vs. Osteopathy (D.O.)

When considering a medical school education, an applicant should be aware of the choice between the allopathic and osteopathic medical philosophies. The allopathic philosophy can be traced to the 6th century B.C. It originally was based upon the belief that disease was due to an imbalance of the body's fluids and therapy should be directed towards correcting this imbalance with drugs. Today's scientific community understands disease better. However, modern allopathic medicine continues to focus on treating the disease rather than the person through medicinal and surgical interventions.

In 1874, Andrew Taylor Still, M.D., founded the osteopathic philosophy of medicine, which treats the person rather than the disease by focusing on the unity of all body parts and the care of patients as whole persons. Dr. Still recognized that the body has the unique ability to heal it self. If one practiced preventive medicine, ate properly, and kept fit, wellness could be achieved. In addition, he felt that the philosophy of focusing on the treatment of illness through the use of medications (which is the basis of allopathy) was often useless and in many instances harmful.

Today osteopathic medicine also includes the use of diagnostic and therapeutic techniques in which physicians use their hands to correct structural and functional problems in the body. The techniques are not regarded as a panacea, but rather are among a number of useful tools that may be employed by the physician to aid the patient. This is not physical therapy, chiropractic or exercise therapy, but a distinctive form of manual medicine. Today there are over 33,000 osteopathic physicians licensed in the United States. Sixty-one percent of these physicians are primary care physicians while thirty-eight percent are involved in the major medical specialties.

In the United States there are over 100 allopathic medical schools distributed over all 50 states. There are 20 osteopathic medical school spread over 20 states. To obtain more information about the osteopathic and allopathic medical schools please refer to the Convenient Resources section below.

The Osteopathic Medical Education

The educational requirements to receive a degree of Doctor of Osteopathy are very similar to those for the allopathic medical education. However, the osteopathic curriculum reflects an underlying emphasis on preventive, family, and community medicine. The first two years of the osteopathic medical training involve learning the basic sciences with some clinical education. The third and fourth years emphasize clinical education through rotations and electives. Throughout the four-year curriculum, students learn to use osteopathic techniques,which include bone manipulation, for diagnosis and treatment of disease, as well as disease prevention. The techniques are based on extensive knowledge of the body's musculoskeletal system. It is believed that a better understanding of this system, which makes up two-thirds of our body mass, provides a better understanding of how an injury or illness in one part of the body can affect another. Osteopathic medical school graduates are required to participate in a one year rotating internship. This is followed by two or more years of residency training. After the residency program, Doctors of Osteopathy work in hospitals, clinics, private offices, nursing homes, and other health care settings.

Convenient Resources

There are many sources which provide detailed information about each allopathic and osteopathic medical school. For allopathic medical schools, I found the AAMC's "**Medical School Admission Requirements (MSAR)**" most helpful. A new edition is published each May and can be found in most public and college libraries. The book is available for $25.00 + $8.00 shipping and handling. The AAMC also offers, "**Minority Student Opportunities in United States Medical Schools**." This book contains information submitted by each medical school to the AAMC concerning admissions, recruitment, support programs, enrichment programs, financial assistance, and educational partnerships. It also contains statistics like the number of first-time applicants, matriculants, and graduates for each school by gender and race/ethnicity. This book is printed every several years and costs $15.00 plus shipping and handling. To obtain a personal copy of either book write to Association of American Medical colleges ATTN: Membership and Publication orders, Department 66, Washington DC 20055; call (202) 828-0416; or visit on the web at https://services.aamc.org/Publications/index.cfm and then search under "browse a topic: applicants"

When considering osteopathy, the American Association of Colleges of Osteopathic Medicine (AACOM) offers an extensive list of publications. One of the easiest to obtain and view is their **Osteopathic Medical College Information Book**. This book is found on the web at http://www.aacom. org/data/cib/index.html, a PDF version can be saved on your computer, or a copy of the book can be ordered and sent to you free of charge by visiting their web site. This resource describes osteopathic medicine as a career, admission requirements, financial aid, description of the curriculum, and contains links to all the osteopathic medical colleges.

Fine Tuning Your Medical School List

As you make a decision on the general type of medical school that will best meet your needs, consider some additional details of importance.

1) Opportunities for scientific research or early exposure to primary / specialty care medicine.
2) Class size.
3) Tuition, fees, and average financial aid packages.
4) Student support services.
5) Availability of a one year enrollment deferment before matriculation.
6) Opportunity for clinical experience during the first two years.
7) Type of curriculum.
8) The requirement of a senior thesis or in-depth mentor-guided project.
9) Availability of elective courses that supplement the basic science or clinical curriculum.
10) Availability of a medical interviewing program
11) Medical schools basic science curriculum at one campus and the clinical curriculum
   at a different campus.

Location

Do not take the location of your medical school lightly. This can be critical to a students success. If you desire to be close to your family, will the location allow convenient travel by airplane or vehicle? Are there safe, inexpensive, culturally sensitive neighborhoods with available apartments for rent or is on campus housing available? Are there appropriate community activities and resources you desire like restaurants, grocery stores, churches, movie theatres, restaurants, health clubs, sporting or musical events, etc? Is parking in the neighborhoods and at the medical school convenient and inexpensive?

Will you be required to have a car to travel in the city, to clinical locations, or around the medical campus? Is the weather appropriate and tolerable for your needs and desires? Does the location provide an affordable cost of living?

Duel Degree Programs

Consideration should also be given to medical schools that offer special degree programs. The Medical Scientist Training Program (MSTP) and the MD – PhD degree programs were developed in recognition of the need for medical scientists trained in both basic and clinical science. Program participants work toward an M.D. and Ph.D. degree over seven years. Potential benefits include a yearly stipend and generous financial aid to cover tuition. Many of these programs are sponsored by the National Institutes of Health. It takes seven years to complete this program. Three years are devoted toward Ph.D. research and four toward the medical studies. Students take a break between their second and third year of medical school to complete the research. Programs are offered in anatomy, biochemistry, biomedical engineering, biophysics, cell biology, genetics, immunology, microbiology, molecular biology, neurosciences, pathology, pharmacology, and physiology. The MD – JD degree program is for students with an interest in medical law. The MD – MBA degree program is for students interested in the business aspect of medicine. The MD – MPH degree program is for students interested in addressing health issues for larger populations. It may take a total of five to six years to finish any of these degree programs. Information about all these degree programs and the allopathic medical schools that offer them can be found at: http://services.aamc.org/currdir/section3/degree2.cfm. Select the appropriate category of interest in the search bar.

Choosing to participate in a duel degree vs. traditional medical school program can be difficult. The additional years of study may seem overwhelming. However, if you have any bit if interest in law, business, or public health this may just be the most convenient opportunity to complete both courses of study. Once you finish your medical education, begin work in the medical field, and develop a family with children, you will have many barriers that would make it difficult to obtain a second degree later in your medical career.

Medical Residency Plans and Career Goals

As you are completing the final stages of college or your post baccalaureate classes, the thought of post-medical school residency training may be far from mind. However, sit back and take a few minutes to consider this stage. Medical residency programs accept more students who graduate from their medical school compared with any other group of applicants. The residency program faculty teach the 3rd and 4th year medical students when they rotate through their department. Over the rotation the faculty become familiar with the student's desire for their specialty, work ethic, ability to work with others, and have the opportunity to assess how well the student works within their system. Knowing this, if you expect to enter a medical profession in which the residency training programs are very competitive, consider choosing a medical school and hospital system with a residency program in that specialty. When you rotate through the department as a 3rd and 4th year medical student, there will be ample opportunity to obtain the necessary exposure for successful admission into that program.

Public vs. Private Medical Schools

An additional area to consider is attending a public medical school in your state of residence or a private medical school. Many publicly supported medical schools favor in state residents and are less expensive to attend. When considering an out of state medical school, carefully compare the number of out of state acceptances to out of state applicants. If the percentage is very low, your chance of acceptance may be small.

Historically Black Medical Schools

Consider one of the nation's historically Black medical schools (**Morehouse School of Medicine** in Atlanta, Georgia; **Meharry Medical College** in Nashville, Tennessee; **Howard University College of Medicine** in Washington, D.C.; and **Charles R. Drew University of Medicine and Science** in Los Angeles, California). These schools have a rich and strong history of producing some of America's most renowned physicians. Having the opportunity to work with other African American and minority students in a relaxing and non-competitive atmosphere can be very enriching. Historically Black medical schools have a large number of minority faculty members compared to most institutions. This can provide plenty of role models and mentors to fit different personalities and career interests. In addition, the curriculum tends to focus on medical problems and issues that pertain to under-represented minorities.

Non-Historically Black Medical Schools

The non-historically Black medical schools can be a good alternative. Because there are more of them, together they offer a larger choice in location, curriculum, clinical opportunities, and duel degree options.

There are several characteristics to assess how receptive the medical school is toward minority students. First, examine the number of minority students enrolled in each class of the medical school and their graduation rate. If the enrollment is large and the graduation rate is excellent, their must be something or someone positive at the school. Often a school offers attractive scholarships, has an exceptional office of minority affairs, provides convenient support services, has active and involved minority faculty members, clinical opportunities with minority populations, active minority medical student organizations like the Student National Medical Association (SNMA), National Network of Latin American Medical Students (NNLAMS), or Association of Native American Medical Students (ANAMS), or an active minority community physician association. When considering these schools, understand that as time goes by scholarship programs are discontinued, people change jobs, and once friendly atmospheres can change. Therefore, do not judge a school by its past but rather by what you expect it will offer over the next four years.

Hispanic Centers of Excellence

Hispanic Centers of Excellence are medical schools who have applied for and received three-year grants from the United States Department of Health and Human services. The grants provide funding to support schools that are committed to train Hispanic students. Participating schools typically offer programs that recruit, train, support, and mentor Hispanic high school, college, and medical school students. Schools also work toward producing physicians who will work in underserved communities and provide special education courses and programs that promote Latino cultural sensitivity. For a list of the 11 participating medical schools, please see the appendix.

Native American Centers of Excellence

The Native American Centers of Excellence are medical schools who have applied for and received three year grants from the United States Department of Health and Human services. The grants provide funding to support schools that are committed to train Native American students. Participating schools typically offer programs that recruit, train, support, and mentor Native American high school, college, and medical school students. Schools also work toward producing physicians who will work in underserved communities and provide special education courses and programs that promote Native American cultural sensitivity. A list of the three participating schools is in the appendix.

Hispanic-Serving Health Professions Schools (HSHPS)

In 1996, the HSHPS was established with support from the US Department of Health and Human Services in response to President Clinton's Executive Order 12900, "Educational Excellence for Hispanic Americans." The Mission is to improve the health of Hispanics through academic development, research initiatives, and training. Currently there are 22 medical school members (please see the appendix for this list).

How Many Medical School Should I Apply To?

While deciding which medical schools are best suited for you, it is also necessary to decide how many you want to apply to. There are no magic numbers: some students choose 5 to 6 schools while others choose 15-20. However, according to the Association of American Medical Colleges the average number of applications to allopathic medical schools submitted by minority medical student applicants in 2001 was 11-12 medical schools.[2]

Early Decision Program

For some students, choosing among the large number of allopathic and osteopathic medical schools is not a concern because they already know what school they want to attend. If you find yourself in a similar situation, you may want to consider applying to medical school under the 'Early Decision Program'. In this program, you have to take the spring MCAT exam and then send in your application shortly after June 15 when the submission period begins. When the medical school receives your application, the admissions committee will review it. The committee can accept, reject, or put the file in the regular decision applicant pool. Early decision applicants are only allowed to apply to one medical school and if accepted they are required to attend that school. If you are not accepted into a medical school through this extremely competitive program then you are free to apply to other medical schools.

This program has a clear advantage. You can get the application and interview process over quickly. Unfortunately, the risk is high. Medical schools need not notify you until October 1st, either of your acceptance/rejection, or your application being placed in the regular applicant pool. If you are not accepted and decide to apply to other medical schools, you still are responsible for submitting all applications before the each school's application deadline. For the most current information about this program, you can go to the internet site: http://www.aamc.org/students/applying/programs/earlydecision. htm.

Below are the allopathic medical schools with the highest total minority student graduates in 2004.

Allopathic Medical Schools with the most Mexican American Graduates in 2004

1. University of Texas Medicine Branch at Galveston
2. University of Texas medical School at San Antonio
3. University of California School of Medicine
4. Baylor College of Medicine
5. University of Texas Medical School at Houston
6. University of New Mexico School of Medicine
7. University of Illinois College of Medicine
8. University of Texas Southwestern Medical Center at Dallas
9. Keck School of Medicine at the University of Southern California
10. Michigan State University College of Human Medicine

Allopathic Medical Schools with the most African American Graduates in 2004

1. Howard University College of Medicine
2. Mehary Medical College
3. Wayne State University School of Medicine
4. Morehouse School of Medicine, Atlanta, Georgia
5. State University of New York Health Science Center Brooklyn College of Medicine
6. Temple University School of Medicine
7. MCP Hahnemann University School of Medicine
8. Medical University of South Carolina
9. University of Tennessee, Memphis College of Medicine
10. University of Michigan Medical School

Allopathic Medical Schools with the most Native American Graduates in 2004

1. University of Oklahoma College of Medicine
2. University of Minnesota Medical School – Twin Cities
3. University of Hawaii John A. Burns School of Medicine
4. Harvard Medical School
5. The Brody School of Medicine of East Carolina University
6. University of North Dakota School of Medicine and Health Sciences
7. Meharry Medical College
8. Uniformed Services University of the Health Sciences
   F. Edward Herbert School of Medicine
9. Medical College of Wisconsin

Mainland Allopathic Medical Schools with the most Puerto Rican Graduates in 2004

1. UMDNJ – New Jersey Medical School
2. Harvard Medical School
3. University of Pennsylvania School of Medicine
4. University of Florida College of Medicine
5. University of Illinois College of Medicine
6. Tufts University School of Medicine
7. UMDNJ- Robert Wood Johnson Medical School
8. Columbia University College of Physicians and Surgeons
9. Baylor College of Medicine
10. Joan & Sanford Weill Medical College of Cornell University
11. New York University School of Medicine
12. State University of New York at Buffalo School of Medicine & Biomedical Sciences
13. Temple University School of Medicine

News Flash!

Medical History Gazette

Vol 1, No 6• The First Source for Medical History •Columbia, S.C.

Dr. Barnes Becomes First Black Physican Admitted to American Board of Otolaryngology

On April 4, 1887, William Henry Barnes was born into a financially strapped family living in Philadelphia, Pennsylvania. As a young boy, he dreamed of becoming a doctor. In spite of being derided by his friends and family for holding such a dream, Dr. Barnes kept his physical energy and spirit focused on achieving his goal.

Graduating in 1908 with a Bachelor of Arts degree, William was determined to continue his studies at the U. of Pennsylvania Medical School. Amid continued negative peer pressure, he studied for and passed the medical school's entrance exam. In fact, his score was so high that the school awarded him a four year scholarship. He graduated four years later; 1912.

Dr. Barnes was appointed as an assistant otolaryngologist at Douglass Hospital in 1913. In 1918 he began serving as an acting assistant surgeon in the U.S. Public Health Service. Continuing his medical education in 1921, Dr. Barnes took post-graduate courses on the ear, nose and throat, as well as special courses on operative surgery at the U. of Pennsylvania. Efforts to

> Dr. Barnes became the first Black physician to limit his practice (specialize) to one area of clinical medicine.

improve his base of knowledge was rewarded when he was promoted to chief Otolaryngologist at Douglass Hospital. In the same year, 1921, he also became a clinical assistant otolaryngologist at Jefferson Medical School's teaching hospital.

Amid much criticism from fellow Black physicians, Dr. Barnes announced in 1922 that he was going to limit his medical practice (specialize) to the ear, nose, and throat. This was a pioneering move at that time since most Black physicians then considered any move toward specialization to be a move toward financial disaster. However, Dr. Barnes was successful in his quest and became the first Black physician to receive certification by the American specialty board of Otolaryngology.

Between 1924 and 1926, Dr. Barnes continued to improve his abilities by studying in France at the U. of Paris in Bordeaux. Under the auspices of Dr. Chevalier Jackson, Dr. Barnes studied the methodology of using the bronchoscope and eventually became the first

See **Specialization** next page

Black physician to master the technique of its use. With this new gift, Dr. Barnes organized and headed a department of Bronchoscopy at Mercy Hospital and was appointed lecturer and consultant in bronchoscopy at Howard U. Medical school.

In spite of an increasingly busy schedule, Dr. Barnes was a progressive innovator. He invented the hypophyscope, used for visualizing the pituitary gland. In addition he devised a variety of medical recording systems and cards containing drawings of the ear, nose, and throat from which pathological changes could be sketched. As a surgeon, he developed and modified many existing techniques.

On a social level, Dr. Barnes was devoted to his family and was deeply religious. On September 21, 1912, he married Miss Mattie E. Thomas. They had five sons of which two pursued and received M.D. degrees. Dr. Barnes regularly attended the Zoar Methodist Church and continually made enough time to be president of the church's board of trustees for over fifteen years. In addition, he was also able to find time to volunteer in his community and became one of the original members of the Philadelphia Housing Authority. Dr. Barnes gained respect and admiration from the Black community for he fought to insure that a just proportion of housing was made available for members of his community.

In 1938, Dr. Barnes began to suffer from hypertension and on January 15, 1945, he died of broncho-pneumonia. Though Dr. Barnes died at an early age, fifty-eight, he had an enormous impact on the field of medicine. In spite of his Black peers continually discouraging him from going beyond the "established" lines of general practice, he persevered. Dr. Barnes is a man we can all look to for inspiration; his life is a truly shining example that failure can only come from within.

Demand for Black Physicians Promotes the Establishment of Black Medical Schools

A few of the early American medical schools would accept Black applicants but a majority did not. And, those schools that did would allow only one to enroll at a time. This was not enough. The Black community needed more Black physicians to care for its health needs.

The first Black medical school opened on November 9, 1868, The Medical Department of Howard University. Eight years later, 1876, Central Tennessee College opened its doors. A year later, Five Irish brothers named Meharry donated $15,000 to the school. For their generous donation the school was renamed Meharry Medical College.

The third Black medical college to open was Leonard Medical School of Shaw University in Raleigh, North Carolina. It opened its doors in 1882 and was the first Black medical school to have a four year curriculum. Six years later, 1888, Louisville National Medical College of Louisville, Kentucky opened its doors. The state legislature granted Dr. Henry Fitzbutler and other local physicians a charter to open the school. Seven other Black medical schools were established from 1889 till 1900.

Howard and Meharry were the only Black medical schools to survive due to poor funding and an inability to keep up with the advances in medical education and technology.

Chapter VII

"You may write me down in history with your bitter, twisted lies. You may throw me in the very dirt but still, like dust I rise."

-Maya Angelou-

The Medical School Application

After taking the MCAT exam, one of the next steps in applying to medical school is completing your medical school application. The application consists of your letters of recommendation, the American Medical College Admissions Service (AMCAS) application and/or the American Association of Colleges of Osteopathic Medicine Application Service (AACOMAS) application, and your transcripts.

Recommendations

Letters of recommendations can be one of the most difficult aspects of the application process. Typically you are required to submit recommendations from two of your science or math professors, and another recommendation from any other person who can attest to your abilities and character, and yet another recommendation from your school's pre-medical committee or advisor. Letters of recommendation can have a significant impact if they describe you in a realistic fashion. Additionally, they should detail your ability to handle both basic and in-depth scientific concepts.

Do not wait until your junior year to establish rapport with your pre-medical advisor and/or committee members. Instead, establish rapport early so that they will have known you at least for a couple of years. Over this time your advisor or committee members will have the opportunity to get to know you and see that you have what it takes to be a medical student and future medical doctor. Though your other recommendations are important it is critical that you receive an exceptional letter from your advisor or committee members.

Getting recommendations from science faculty members can be difficult, especially if your classes are large and do not facilitate direct interaction with the professor. If you anticipate such a situation, make an effort to go to your course professors within the first few days of class and frequently thereafter. Even if you do not have many questions pertaining to class, go anyway. Let your professors know who you are, and give them time to let you know a little bit about who they are, what they have done, and where they are going. Establishing this contact early will be valuable when it is time to ask for a recommendation. Not only will the professor have more of an interest in writing the recommendation, but will know enough about you that the recommendation can come from personal experience.

Often in large classes, there are a number of teaching assistants and/or lab instructors. If you end up connecting with the assistants more than the course instructor do not hesitate to ask for a recommendation. In my genetics course, I often went to my lab instructor for help. Over the course of the semester, she became my unofficial tutor and personal genetics mentor. As the semester matured, she was able to watch me struggle with material yet in the end do very well in the course. Asking her for a recommendation was a natural step for me because she personally knew my dedication, skill, and ability to work hard.

Do not be anxious about asking a professor for a recommendation in a particular course in which you weren't a superior student but still worked very hard to get a respectable grade. Professor's notice the students who work hard and ask good questions. They will be able to attest to the fact that you work hard and do not give up when a class is difficult.

If you intimately worked with a professor during your freshman or sophomore year do not wait till the second semester of your junior year to ask that professor for a recommendation. Rather immediately request the letter and have the professor send the recommendation to your pre-medical advisor who can put it in your folder. As time passes, your stellar academic performance may fade from the professor's memory and when the second semester of your junior year rolls around you may be just another student that took his or her course. If after taking other courses, you receive better recommendations your pre-medical advisor will be able to choose the strongest letters of recommendation for you.

Some of you will not have the opportunity to establish a good working relationship with many of your science or math professors. Then you must determine the course(s) in which you did the best, and go to that professor and request a written recommendation. You may feel awkward doing this because this professor might not know you very well. However, the professor will know their course, and can attest to the fact that you are academically capable of handling similar material in medical school. To help the professor(s) write a positive recommendation, provide them with a resume or curriculum vitae (CV) and a copy of your personal essay that you will submit with the AMCAS application. This will give the professor extra information to personalize your letter of recommendation.

If you intend to ask some of your professors for recommendations during the second semester of your junior year, go to them as early as possible. They are less likely to turn down early requests. In addition, an early request provides the professor with plenty of time to write a quality recommendation. When you ask a professor for a recommendation be sure that you ask in a friendly but direct manner if he/she will be able to write a letter that is, without qualification, completely positive. Having made it this far the last thing you need is a negative recommendation.

Each time a professor agrees to write a recommendation, send a thank you letter a week or two later. This will serve as a pleasant reminder of their agreement. If you subsequently win a special award or complete a project in which you are honored, let the recommender(s) know. Such information can only enhance your recommendation.

A great source for the non-science/math recommendation is a supervisor with whom you worked during a summer program. Having worked with this individual for an entire summer, not only will they know a little bit about you, but they will also be able to attest to your character and other personal qualities.

One last bit of information. At some point during the application process, you will be asked whether you will waive your legal right to see the letters of recommendation that are submitted by your pre-medical committee to each medical school you choose to apply. Though there is no indication that not waiving your rights will hurt your chances for admission to medical school, some may use it against you. As an applicant you should know that each recommendation is positive.

The AMCAS/AACOMAS Application

Admissions officers representing many of America's medical schools came together and organized an admissions service that simplifies and standardizes the process of applying to medical school. The process begins with your submitting an application to the admissions service. The admissions service then processes the material and sends a complete copy to each medical school on the list you supply them.

The application asks you to provide information from nine major areas:

1. Biographical;
2. List of colleges, graduate and professional schools attended;
3. Honors received;
4. Extracurricular, community, and vocational activities;
5. Employment during school years (list type of work and approx. hours per week);
6. What you have done during your summer vacation while in college;
7. If you have taken time off from school and what you did;
8. Personal essay (AMCAS application only);
9. Academic record (Transcripts from all colleges, graduate, and professional schools attended).

The best strategy for submitting the application is to be organized and begin early. You can do this by opening a résumé in your computer files your first year of college, and begin entering each new item, relative to those first six areas, as it becomes available. Say you win an award your first year of college, or transfer to another school, or complete a summer activity; enter this information immediately. Keep this up through college. When it is time to complete the application everything you need will be at your fingertips (See the appendix for a sample résumé).

The AMCAS and AACOMAS application can only be completed on-line. Familiarize yourself with the two programs by visiting the American Association of Medical Colleges web site at http://www.aamc.org/students/amcas/start.htm or visit the American Association of Colleges of Osteopathic Medicine website at https://aacomas.aacom.org/. It is imperative to read all the accompanying instructions carefully and thoroughly. The application can be very confusing, especially the academic record section. If you have trouble, do not worry, you are not the only one. Seek help immediately from your pre-medical advisor.

On the application, you may not be able to include all the information you would like. Prioritize your information and include that which is most important and will best highlight the application. Eliminate words and phrases that are unnecessary. If there is information you left off the application, do not forget about it. You may have the opportunity to include it on your secondary application.

The personal essay is the part of the AMCAS application where you get to write about anything you want. It may be about your reason for wanting to become a doctor, a short biography, a medical experience you have had, etc. Again, space will be limited. Before you begin your essay be sure you check and see how long it can be. Though your space may be limited, look to write a concise and creative essay for the space you do have. Also, be sure to write your essay before it is time for you to actually complete the application. After you have created your personal essay give it to an English professor, a fellow student, and/or bring it to a writing center if your school offers one. Have your essay read over and get feedback. Most students take at least a month or more to generate the final draft. In the appendix, there are ten sample essays written by minority students who attended medical school. Use them as a topic and creativity guide for your own essay.

As with the other sections of the application, completing the academic record section tends to be difficult due to the limited space available. One method for easing this problem is to have a copy of your transcript(s) and use the course title abbreviations used on the transcript. This way you will not have to create your own abbreviations and as the academic record and the transcript are reviewed there will be no discrepancies that could delay the processing of the application.

If multiple academic institutions have been attended, obtaining transcripts can be difficult when you are no longer at the institution. With this in mind, before you leave each institution write down in a safe place the phone number and address of each school's transcript office. Many transcript offices will not process a transcript request unless a request with an original signature has been received.

When the application is finished, print a copy for your records. This record can be referenced in case of difficulties. Maintaining a copy of the personal essay can be an asset during interviews. Many interviewers will ask questions specifically about topics from the essay.

Submitting Your Application

It is important to complete the application early. Applications completed at the earliest acceptable time will be processed first and without delay. The application service tends to process a large number of applications from the end of July to the end of August. During this time it takes longer to process applications.

When you submit your application early, the application service will be able to quickly notify you if there are any missing materials or other problems which will prevent the application from being processed. If the application is submitted during the peak time or later it may take an extended period of time before you are informed of the problem. If this occurs, you have little time to make the correction and your application to a particular medical school can potentially be jeopardized.

The Patient

They come to you from all walks of life.
Rich and Poor,
Young and Old,
Men, Women, and Children.

They arrive
Vulnerable and defenseless.

They share their most inner thoughts,
Cares and concerns,
Aches and pains,
Life experiences revealed only to you.

They are asked
To expose their most sacred possession: their bodies.

They listen to your words
Of advice and counsel,
Reassurance and guidance,
Direction and education.

They follow your instructions because
You are trusted,
An advocate for their needs.

They are called the patient
And you are the physician

News Flash!

Medical History Gazette

Vol 1, No 7• The First Source for Medical History •Columbia, S.C.

Ohiyesa (Charles Eastman)
An American Indian Physician

Ohiyesa, was born in 1858 in Southwestern Minnesota. His parents were of the Dakota nation. His mother died several months after he was born and his paternal grandmother, Uncheeda, raised him.

In 1862, there was the Minnesota Dakota conflict and Ohiyesa's father, Jacob "Many Lightings" Eastman, was captured and sent to federal prison. Ohiyesa's family fled the Dakota Territory into Southeastern Manitoba (Canada) where they lived on his uncle's farm. This experience gave him a firm foundation of the life, language, culture, and oral history of his people.

Eleven years later, Ohiyesa's father was released from prison on a pardon by President Lincoln. He traveled to Canada and rejoined his family. The family traveled back to the United States and settled in Flandreau, South Dakota.

With the support of his father, who converted to Christianity while in jail, Ohiyesa was baptized and given the name Charles Alexander Eastman. He then attended the Flandreau Santee Normal Indian School.

An outstanding student, Charles graduated and matriculated to Knox College and then transferred to Dartmouth College. At school he played football, ran track, played tennis, boxing, and baseball. Academically he chose to pursue a career in medicine. He graduated in 1886 and then entered the medical school of Boston College. He graduated in June 1889 and became one of the first Native American men to receive a medical degree.

Dr. Eastman, returned to South Dakota to work for the Bureau of Indian Affairs and was assigned to the Pine Ridge Agency.

In December 1890, tension was brewing in the area. Members of the local Sioux Indian nation had lost their ability to move freely. Instead they were confined to reservations where they were dependent on the reservation administrators.

A new hope rose in the community that the Sioux would rise again to glory. This hope was expressed in the ghost dance. The administrative agents in Pine Ridge grew worried and obtained orders to arrest Chief Sitting Bull, the Sioux leader. He was killed on December 15, 1890.

Chief Big Foot took over and proceeded to lead his people toward the Pine Ridge Indian Reservation. On December 29, 1890, the local army was dispatched, captured the group, and

See **Ohiyesa** next page

Ohiyesa: Continued from previous page

brought them to the banks of Wounded Knee creek. Eventually shots rang out and when the smoke cleared approximately 300 Sioux men, women, and children and 25 soldiers were killed. Some of the wounded were brought to Dr. Eastman who attended to their medical needs. The next day, despite a freezing blizzard, Dr. Eastman was the first physician to reach Wounded Knee. He discovered a few survivors among the carnage of battle.

Dr. Eastman had seen enough corruption and thievery of reparation money and now the killing of his fellow Indians. His protests came upon deaf ears and he left Pine Ridge in 1893.

His family moved to St. Paul, Minnesota. He passed the licensing exam and began to practice medicine. However, constant harassment by local physicians and authorities prevented him from being able to provide medical care.

In 1900, he and his family moved to South Dakota where he was appointed to provide medical care for the Crow Creek Agency. His continued efforts to support and stand up for his fellow Indian led to his firing a year later.

After 1902, Dr. Eastman became an accomplished author. He wrote about the American Indian culture with the hope that it would provide greater understanding and bring greater respect to his people. His writings included autobiographical works, children's stories, and works of philosophy.

Dr. Eastman participated in many projects. This included supporting a summer camp for girls, traveling on a lecture tour, and serving on the Committee of One Hundred to advise President Coolidge on Indian policy.

In recognition of his work, Dr. Eastman was presented a special medal at the 1933 Chicago World's Fair for providing the most distinguished achievements by an American Indian. Dr. Eastman died in 1939.

Dr. Numa P. G. Adams:
First African American Dean of a US Medical School

Numa P. G. Adams was born on February 26, 1885 in Delaplane, Virginia. At a young age he became quite close to his grandmother, Mrs. Amanda Adams. He particularly enjoyed assisting his grandmother in dispensing medicinal herbs to the residents of the community.

After graduating from high school with honors, Numa served as a public school teacher. Two years later, he entered Howard University and graduated magna cum laude. The following year he was awarded a masters degree, in chemistry, from Columbia University.

From there he became an entry-level chemistry teacher and was able to quickly work his way up. Seven years after he began, he was selected to become head of the chemistry department.

Numa decided to change the focus of his career by enrolling at Rush Medical College located in Chicago, Illinois on March 29, 1920. Continuing a tradition begun at Howard, Numa earned his living at night as a musician while he went to school during the day. Such a demanding schedule did not affect his academic

See **Dean** next page

performance, for on February 13, 1925, Dr. Adams was licensed to practice medicine as a surgeon in the state of Illinois.

In 1927 Howard University College of Medicine was in a state of transition. Major efforts were being made to bring the medical school up to the standards established by the majority medical institutions. Part of the transition lay in the selection of a new dean. Most people affiliated with the medical school believed a ranking white doctor would be given the position. However, Howard's president, Dr. Mordecai W. Johnson had a different idea and hired Dr. Numa Adams making him the first African American to be dean of an accredited medical school in the United States.

When Dr. Adams became the dean in 1929, he inherited a school that needed major reorganization. The faculty needed to be strengthened, the curriculum reorganized, the affiliation between Freedman's hospital and the medical school needed clarification and new lines of authority and responsibility had to be designated, funding had to be found to support the changes, the admissions standards had to be raised, and a positive working environment for students and faculty had to be developed.

It was not long before Dr. Adams' ideas and methods to reorganize the medical school were met with anger and resentment. Everyday was a struggle and a fight for him. However, he met the challenge and was able to develop Howard University College of Medicine into a nationally respected medical school.

During his tenure, he was able to secure Freedman's Hospital as the schools primary teaching hospital. He pushed his new recruits to work toward their Ph.D.'s and encouraged them to travel to different parts of the country and pursue the most successful research labs. Dr. Adams pushed his clinical faculty members to get the best continuing training possible.

Faculty members encountered problems because most hospitals would not accept Black doctors into their programs. Thus, he brought two distinguished white physicians to the school of medicine. He had them organize and develop the department of surgery of which Dr. Charles R. Drew became head five years later.

To raise the quality of students accepted to the medical school, Dr. Adams reduced the class size. Against popular opinion it was his belief that quality was infinitely more important than quantity; "Howard's doctors are going to be first rate physicians". The last four years of his deanship; no student failed the state board examination, a feat never to be repeated.

Though Dr. Adams was able to create a positive change in such a short time while also raising the medical school to national respectability, little praise was forthcoming from his colleagues. He received no honorary degrees, medals of honor, certificates of merit, achievement awards, or posts of salute. In spite of this, he was able to keep his motivation and spirit alive with the satisfaction of seeing the seeds he planted begin to grow and flourish.

However, the many battles and extensive obligations slowly began to affect Dr. Adams' health. He died at the age of fifty-five, August 29, 1940, during his eleventh year as dean of Howard University College Of Medicine.

Since Dr. Adams' death, his efforts and work at the Howard University College of Medicine have become appreciated. Dr. Joseph L. Johnson, Dean of the medical school in 1951, commented that, "He was of brilliant mind and was always the quiet, unassuming, soft-spoken gentleman. One could never know of his greatness from his lips."

Chapter VIII

Medical School Admissions

Admission committees are principally composed of faculty members from basic science and clinical departments. Frequently there are one or more medical student members. At a few schools, the committees include faculty members from other colleges and universities in the area.

Processing of Applications

When a medical school receives an application, the admissions committee will screen it and determine if the applicant meets the schools standard for academic quality. An applicant who meets this standard is sent a secondary application or is contacted to arrange an interview.

The secondary application varies between schools. Some schools only request basic biographical information while other schools require you to write an essay(s). It is important to note that many of the osteopathic medical schools request that the student submit a letter of recommendation from an osteopathic physician. Applicants who continue to meet the school's usual standards for academic quality are contacted by the admissions office to arrange an interview.

In the event the secondary application is returned in a timely fashion but there is no response from the medical school, call the admissions office. Explain the situation to the receptionist. Some applications are misplaced, misfiled, and even lost.

Selection Factors

It is difficult to specify the exact criteria each school uses to determine who is selected for an interview. It is safe to say that most medical schools do not seek a stereotyped ideal combination of characteristics in their applicants. Diversity within an entering class is very desirable. Though there is no academic cut off, committees often give priority to students who have demonstrated a high level of scholastic achievement and show exceptional academic potential in medical school. Typically this is evaluated by reviewing the grades from the pre-medical classes, the lettes of recommendations, MCAT scores, and any special program, projects, or experience .

The Interview Season

At most medical schools the interview season begins in September and ends in April. The students who complete and send in their applications early and quickly return the secondary applications tend to obtain the best interview dates.

The medical school admissions system is set up so that a student who interviews in September and October has the same opportunity as a student who interviews during March and April. However, this is not the case. Most medical schools accept their students for admission on a "rolling basis". This means that during the interview season the admissions committee will meet about every two weeks. All the applicants interviewed during that two-week period will have their files and interviews presented to the committee for consideration. The admission's committee will accept the applicant for admission, deny the applicant for admission, or put the application in a file for reconsideration at a later date. Applicants are notified of the committee's decision. Applicants who receive a letter of admission are given about two weeks to accept or decline the offer.

Even though an applicant accepts a schools offer for admission, they are still able to interview and receive admission to other medical schools. Thus, an applicant can hold multiple admission spots. Often, "the dust clears" in early May. At this time, applicants who have multiple acceptances have to choose the school they intend to matriculate. Because of the medical school's "rolling admissions" policy and an applicants ability to hold multiple admissions spots, medical school's are forced to accept two to three times as many applicants as they expect to matriculate.

Early in the interview season, each school's pool of accepted applicants who are holding a spot is quite small. Therefore, the admission's committee is more liberal in sending out letters of acceptance. However, towards the end of the interview season the pool of accepted applicants who are holding a spot is quite large. Admissions committee's fear that if too many students receive acceptance letters, the class could be too large. Therefore, applicants who interview late in the season are less likely to receive a letter of acceptance but rather are placed on a wait list. Once the "dust clears" after the early May deadline, medical schools have a better look at their class size. If more students are needed, then additional letters of acceptance are mailed to the applicants who remain on the waiting list.

Scheduling Your Interview & Preparing for the Visit

Each medical school that selects an applicant for an interview will send a letter requesting them to schedule a time to visit. Again, an applicant who is selected for an interview early in the season will find that each school's interview schedule is wide open and will be able to schedule the interview at a time that is convenient to the applicant rather then just the school.

Great care should be taken when scheduling interviews. For example, if you have applied to some medical schools that are close together, arrange your schedule so all the interviews can be completed in one trip. Multiple trips are costly and disrupt your college courses. As well, those interviews that require significant travel should be scheduled as early in the fall as possible. Once winter sets in, the weather can be very unpredictable and often there are travel delays. The last thing you need is to miss an interview to your favorite medical school because of a snowstorm.

Once your interview schedule is set, take time and prepare for the visits. Purchase a quality suit or outfit; the more conservative the better. Also, keep in mind the cooler weather of the fall and winter. Consider purchasing a quality suitcase that you can carry on a plane; the last thing you need is a lost suitcase. Be sure you have excellent directions and double-check your dates and times. Carry important medical school phone numbers in the event your trip encounters problems. Don't forget to bring a copy of any application information and essays submitted to the school for last minute reference. The night before your vist go to bed early so you are well rested. The interview day can be draining and you want to be your best the entire time.

Your Interview

Each medical school conducts its interview day differently. However, the day will likely begin at the Admissions office. Often you will meet other candidates who have come for an interview. Always be cordial and friendly. One of them may be your next classmate. From there you will meet members of the admissions staff and administration. You will have a tour of the medical school and its facilities. If the teaching hospital is near you may also walk through it. Lunch is often included in your visit. Many schools use this as a time for you to meet some of the current medical students. Take this opportunity to ask questions.

Finally your interview. Rarely is their just one. But rather, a combination with a faculty member, a medical student, and the director of admissions. Some schools will have an applicant interview with two or more people at one time.

During the day you will meet many people. Consider carrying a small notepad to write down the names of important faculty, administration, and students. This can be a great reference in the future.

The Interview: What Do They Want to Find Out?

The universal opinion is that medicine demands superior personal attributes of its students and practitioners. Integrity and responsibility assume major importance in the research laboratory, classroom, and with patients and colleagues. Personal attributes medical schools look for include leadership, communication skills, maturity, diverse personal interests (educational, social, cultural), high degree of concern for people, social maturity and emotional stability, initiative, curiosity, common sense, perseverance, personal motivation, and the ability to work within a team setting. The purpose of the interview is to give the interviewer a chance to see that you have these qualities. The interview also gives the interviewer the opportunity to ask questions about parts of your application that may present questions. For instance, if there was a science class in which you received a low grade or a section on the MCAT exam in which you did not score particularly well.

Before your interview, the interviewer may review your application and essay so they know a little about you. With this in mind, it is a good idea to review your application and personal essay before the interview. Don't be caught off guard. In many cases, however, the interviewer has not had time to review your application or has a policy of not doing so before interviews. Either way you should feel comfortable discussing a wide range of issues and topics.

Some of the more popular open-ended interview questions include:
1. "Why do you want to be a doctor?"
2. "Tell me about yourself."
3. "If you were in situation 'X', what would you do?"

In addition, be ready for such detailed questions as:
4. "How did you study for your last midterm or final exam?"
5. "Tell me about a patient who you have interacted with that has made an impact on you?"
6. "What value or values have you taken from your mother and/or father? "
        (See the appendix for an extensive list of interview questions)

During the interview, the interviewer is probably going to ask you which field of medicine you like the most. This question is used to assess how long you have actually been considering the medical field. in addition, it lets the interviewer know what medical interests you have; research, primary care medicine, or a high level specialty. Many medical schools tend to accept those students who have medical interests that coincide with those of the school. Thus, if you are interested in family medicine, your chances of acceptance at a research institution are less but greater at a medical school emphasizing primary care medicine.

The interviewer may also ask why you chose to apply to their medical school. In preparation for this question, it is important to contemplate why you selected that school. Was it because of a particular department, early clinical experience, its record of accomplishment for graduating medical students who choose to specialize in particular fields, location close to family and friends.

During the interview you may find that very little of the conversation is about medicine. Instead, the conversation may be about foreign films, literature, travels, music, or some other topic which you indicated on your application. As a result, don't lie on your application because you may be required to demonstrate, perform, or otherwise prove that you have had the experience, training, or ability. In addition, do not get discouraged or feel that you were in some way inadequate if the discussion was not about your medical interests or your application. This situation often may indicate that after reviewing your application the interviewer already believes you are academically qualified to attend their school. Instead, the interviewer's goal is to assess if you have the right type of personality and character that fits the schools own personality and character.

Remember that if the interviewer asks a question you feel is unreasonable, you do not have to answer the question. Areas of unreasonable questioning include your plans for a family, or any racial, religious, gender, or sexual preferences. However, if you included the topic in the application the interviewer has the right to inquire about it.

The Interview: What Do You Want to Find Out?

Often when we are caught up in the excitement of being selected for an interview, we forget that the interview is also our chance to decide whether we really like the school. I have found that the only true way to know what a school is like is to stay with a medical student. With your notification of interview selection, some schools will inform you of the option to stay with a minority medical student. If this occurs, jump at the opportunity. If a medical school does not indicate such a program exists, take the time to call the school's admissions office and inquire about staying with a minority medical student. Often the admissions staff will be happy to work something out for you.

In considering this option, ask to stay with a second year medical student. These students have had more time to interact with the administration, the community, and really understand the curriculum. If you interview early, the 1st year medical students may have had only a couple of months of medical school experience.

When you stay with a minority student, you will have a greater opportunity to interact with other minority students. Thus, you will be able to get a broad range of opinions about the school. Some medical schools may be in transition or major issues may be floating around creating an uncertain academic climate. You most likely will only learn of these issues by talking to the students. In addition, your host will be able to give you a good sense of the community in which the school is located and how well it will fit your taste and personal interests. As I will discuss later in 'financing a medical education', there is also a great economic benefit of staying with a medical student.

While you are at the medical school do not be afraid to talk to the students and most importantly, ask questions. Remember, asking questions is especially important during your interview. At some point, the interviewer will give you the opportunity to ask them questions. Use this time to ask some hard and detailed questions. This will demonstrate to the interviewer that you are interested in and seriously considering their medical school. (For a list of questions you can ask, see appendix: Questions To Ask During The Medical School Interview.)

After the Interview

When you get home, it is very courteous to send a thank you letter to your medical school interviewer. If after your visit to the school you decide that this school is everything you are looking for and that if accepted you will matriculate, let the interviewer and the admission's committee know. Sometimes a committee is more likely to accept a student if they are certain the student will matriculate to the school. If nothing else, such letters will force the admissions office to find your application and put the letter with your other materials. Such activity will make sure that your folder was not inadvertently put in the wrong pile or even misplaced; this too has happened before. Also if you receive an award, special designation, or any other achievement after your interview, be sure to inform all the medical schools you are seriously considering. Any new information may be just what is needed to convince the admissions committee that you should be a member of their next medical school class.

Ask, Seek, Knock:

The heart of a Physician

is that of a life long learner.

News Flash!

Medical History Gazette

Vol 1, No 8• The First Source for Medical History •Columbia, S.C.

Dr. Hector P. Garcia:
A Fight to Break Down Barriers

With seven children to care for, Jose and Faustina Garcia fled the Mexican Revolution of 1910-1920 and settled in Mercedes, Texas. Life was hard and the family struggled to survive poverty, segregation, and limited employment opportunities for Mexicans.

The Garcia children was led by a strong willed father who taught them all he learned in school and inspired them with stories about the Aztecs. Hector followed his father's dream for the children and earned a degree at Edinburgh Junior College. He then went on to the University of Texas Medical School in Galveston. He graduated in 1940. Following medical school, Dr. Garcia traveled to Nebraska for his internship (Texas hospitals refused to accept a Mexican American physician).

Dr. Garcia participated in the "Civilian Military Training Corps" and eventually earned an officer's commission. World War II came and many Mexicans, like Dr. Garcia, signed up to fight. Upon his return, he had earned a Bronze star, six Battle Stars, and the rank of Major. The patriotism exhibited was returned with social, economic, and political discrimination.

Dr. Garcia did not back down. In March 1948, he organized the American GI Forum of the United States of America. Its goal was to improve benefits and health care for Mexican American veterans. The group forged alliances with key entertainment and political figures and fought discrimination through the courts. All this activity helped publicize the plight of Mexican Americans. courtroom victories helped break down some of the barriers.

Through Dr. Garcia's successful work and the relationships he built, he was asked to serve on the United States Commission on Civil Rights. Also, President Lyndon B. Johnson appointed him as an alternate Ambassador to the United Nations.

As much as Dr. Garcia was a civil rights leader, he was also known to be just as devoted to medicine and his patients. He practiced medicine in Corpus Christi, Texas.

In 1984, President Regan awarded Dr. Garcia the Presidential Medal of Freedom, the highest civilian award given by the President.

In July 1996, Dr. Garcia died in Corpus Christi, Texas.

> Dr. Garcia was awarded the Presidential Medal of Freedom: The highest civilian honor bestowed by a President

Chapter IX

Financially Surviving The Medical School Application Process

O ne of the most stressful components of the medical school application process is figuring out how to finance ones way. It seems as though the medical school application process is based on a physician's budget and not a college student's budget. However, with this in mind, one must realize there is no way to get into medical school other than by paying the financial dues. Be encouraged, if enough preparation is made, the expenses can be reduced significantly.

Preparing for the MCAT Exam

The commercial preparatory programs tend to be expensive. Stanley Kaplan courses are over $1100 while Princeton Review Inc. tends to be even more expensive. These programs tend to be located on or near college campuses in large metropolitan cities. Some colleges and universities have programs set up to allow their students to take the course at a discounted price. Check with your pre-medical advisor to see if your school gives you this benefit. If not, Stanley Kaplan and Princeton Review Inc. may provide financial aid. The amount of financial aid you will receive is based on the percent of financial aid you receive from your college or university.

The least expensive method of preparing for the MCAT is to purchase a review book. These books tend to cost about $50.00 new. A search on Amazon.com or other internet sources might link you to the same books at less expensive prices. There is also the MCAT practice exams offered by AAMC, as described in Chapter V 'Medical College Admission Test'; each costs $40. Again, the paper exams may be ordered at the following address: ATTN: Membership and Publication Orders, Department 66, Washington DC 20055; call (202) 828-0416; or visit on line at https://services.aamc.org/Publications/index.cfm and under "browse a topic" click on applicants. If you go "online", you will have access to the web based exams as well.

Taking the MCAT Exam

The fee for taking the MCAT exam in 2006 is $210.00. A fee reduction program is available. This will provide aid to individuals with extreme financial limitations. For more information about this program, visit www.aamc.org/fap. Determination of one's ability to pay takes into consideration the student and their parent's income, assets, and expenses as well as liabilities, number of dependent children, number of children in college, graduate school, and professional school. The MCAT fee reduction program will reduce the MCAT testing fee from $210 to $85. Applications for this program are usually due about two months prior to the examination. To participate in the fee reduction program, it is important to be prepared. All required information can be obtained from all financial aid documents and tax statements.

Be aware that you have to apply for the fee reduction program and be approved before an application is sent in for the MCAT exam. A fee reduction approval card must be submitted with the application. Of special note, if the application to the fee reduction program for the MCAT is accepted, the student will automatically qualify for an AMCAS fee waiver if both applications are submitted in the same calendar year.

AMCAS Application

Like the MCAT exam, the AMCAS application is also expensive. In 2006, the fee for the first school chosen is $160.00 and an additional $30.00 for each subsequent school. AMCAS offers a fee assistance program to individuals with extreme financial limitations whose inability to pay the AMCAS service fee would severely inhibit application to medical school. To be eligible for fee assistance, applicants must meet certain gross income requirements based upon family size. Visit on line at www. aamc.org/fap for more information about this program. Again, if you qualified for a fee reduction of the MCAT exam you will qualify for fee assistance with the AMCAS application. If accepted, you are allowed to apply to eleven AMCAS-participating schools without paying the AMCAS service fee.

AACOMAS Application

The AACOMAS services are also expensive. The application fee starts at $155.00 for one school and increase by $20.00 to $35.00 for each successive school. The AACOMAS does offer a fee waiver program. You may be eligible if your annual income level is within the U.S. Bureau of Census low income threshold for a family of your size. A fee wavier can only be applied to a maximum of four osteopathic medical schools. A service fee is required to apply to additional schools. To apply for a fee waiver, contact your school's financial aid office and request that they have the GAPSFAS program send a "Summary of Applicant's Resources" (SOAR) to AACOMAS. In completing the GAPSFAS application be sure that the AACOMAS code number 7363 is designated. For complete information visit: https://aacomas.aacom.org/.

Secondary Applications

After a medical school has reviewed your application, they will usually send you a secondary application. Some schools ask for additional academic or biographical material. However, all schools ask for a secondary application fee. This fee tends to range between $30 and $50 dollars. It is possible to get a fee waiver from each medical school, but in order to do so, you will have to call the admissions office of each school and inquire about the application procedure. Most schools will require a letter from a financial aid officer at your school. In the event you receive an AMCAS fee waiver, make copies of the award letter and mail it with your secondary applications and a cover letter requesting a fee waiver. If you receive a fee waiver from the AACOMAS, the application service will forward your name to the osteopathic colleges you are applying to.

Interviewing

Interviewing is the most expensive aspect of medical school admission. Each medical school wants to meet their applicants and conduct an interview. To do this there are expenses for transportation, food, and accommodations. Though it is impossible to get around paying airfares to travel across the country, it is still possible to save money. If two medical schools are relatively close together, schedule the interviews so you can visit both schools but make only one trip. If some of the medical schools are near your home consider scheduling the interviews over winter break and driving to each school. Be aware that some airlines have special discounts of about 15% - 25% for students flying specifically for graduate and professional school interviews. Some airlines, such as Southwest Airlines, also have special youth fares for people who have not reached their 22nd birthday. A valid picture I.D. is needed to take advantage of this offer. When reservations are made be sure to ask about discounts because they often are not advertised.

One area in which you can be certain of saving money is by staying with a minority student rather than at a hotel. Besides the numerous benefits, as described in the section 'Interview: What Do I Want To Find Out?', taking this initiative will also save money. Some medical schools have organized programs that allow applicants to stay with medical students; others do not. If you do not automatically receive any information about such a program, contact the admissions office. Often, arrangements can be made. It is important to give the admissions office advance notice so they will be able to have the best chance to organize your stay. If you stay with a student, understand that his/her time is very limited. Therefore be certain that you arrive when you say you will. In addition, limit your stay with the student to one or two nights.

Acceptance Deposit

Upon admission to an allopathic medical school, the applicant will have about two weeks to accept or reject the offer. If the offer is accepted, a $100 dollar refundable deposit is submitted to the school. When the applicant matriculates to the school, the deposit is credited toward the fall tuition.

Applicants can hold multiple medical school acceptances by submitting a deposit to each school. Once a decision is made not to attend a school the admission office needs to be contacted and the deposit will be returned. Medical schools expect a final decision to be made by May 15. After that date schools are not required to return the deposit.

Of the osteopathic medical schools only the University of Medicine and Dentistry of New Jersey School of Osteopathic Medicine requires an acceptance deposit. This deposit is refundable until June first.

Problems often arise when applicants fail to prepare for the acceptance deposit. It is exciting to receive acceptance to a large number of schools. However, holding multiple acceptances can be very expensive. With this in mind, prioritize your medical schools. If your first medical school acceptance is to a school that is low on your list and later on you receive an acceptance to a school that is high on your list, ask the lower priority school to return your deposit. Not only will this strategy help financially, but it will help someone else who is eagerly hoping to fill the spot you vacate.

Attributes of a Great Physician

The great physicians of the world

are known for their love, joy, peace, patience,

kindness, goodness, faithfulness, gentleness, and self-control.

Medical History Gazette

Vol 1, No 9• The First Source for Medical History •Columbia, S.C.

News Flash!

Dr. Charles R. Drew leads the way in Blood Banking Project

Charles Drew was born on June 3, 1904 in the northwest section of Washington D.C. commonly known as "Foggy Bottom". When Charles was 10, his family moved to Arlington, Virginia. As the new kid in the neighborhood, Charles had to be strong, self-reliant, and industrious in order to establish himself among the other boys. This proved to be worthwhile for at the age of twelve he established his own newspaper route and eventually had six boys working for him.

In elementary and high school, Charles showed athletic excellence as a member of the football, basketball, and track teams. He was honored twice as the best all round athlete. Graduating from Dunbar High School in 1922, Charles continued his education at Amherst College where he was awarded a partial athletic scholarship. At Amherst, Charles continued to show athletic excellence on the schools football and track teams. In his senior year, he was awarded the Honorable Mention-All American honors as an All Eastern half-back in football.

After graduating from Amherst College in 1926, Charles chose to continue his education

by attending medical school. However, he had to postpone his medical education for two years so he could save money to pay for tuition. During those two years, he taught biology and chemistry at Morgan College located in Baltimore, Maryland while also serving as director of the schools athletic program.

Charles Drew aspired to attend Howard University College of Medicine in Washington, D.C. He was denied admission because he had not satisfied the school's English requirement. Denied admission to Howard, Charles attended McGill University School of Medicine (Montreal, Canada) which had less stringent English admission requirements.

Though in medical school, Charles joined the university's track team and won the high jump, high and low hurdles, and broad jump events at the Canadian Track and Field Championships.[3] Charles Drew's outstanding athletic talent, however, did not overshadow his academic talent for he was one of the top graduating students in his medical school class, was elected to the Alpha Omega

> Dr. Drew was awarded the Doctor of Medical Science degree becoming the first African-American recipient of the degree and he became an expert on any matter dealing with the preservation of blood.

See **Drew** next page

Drew: Cont. from previous page

Alpha, which is a medical honorary scholastic fraternity, and he was awarded the Williams Prize which is given to the student that scores the highest on a competitive examination given to the top five students in the graduating class.

Two years after graduating from medical school, Dr. Drew returned to the United States and became a pathology instructor at Howard University School of Medicine and its affiliated medical center, Freedmen's Hospital. The following year he became an assistant in surgery on the medical school faculty and a surgical resident in Freedmen's hospital. Continuing his rise within the profession, he became an instructor in surgery and assistant surgeon in just his third year at the school and hospital.

As one of the most promising surgical instructors at Howard, Dr. Drew was selected to participate in a faculty development advanced training program. Dr. Drew left Howard and participated in research in the Department of Surgery at Columbia University College of Physicians and Surgeons and as a resident in surgery in Presbyterian Hospital. At the hospital Dr. Drew researched blood preservation. At the completion of the blood preservation research, Dr. Drew was awarded the Doctor of Medical Science degree becoming the first African-American recipient of the degree and an expert on any matter dealing with the preservation of blood.

Dr. Drew returned to Howard University with the goal of producing outstanding African American surgeons. However, his time at Howard as assistant professor of surgery and surgeon at Freedmen's Hospital was cut short.

In 1940 Germany was systematically bombing England causing a large number of causalities and a need for large supplies of plasma. Under the auspices of the Blood Transfusion Association, the "Blood for Britain" project was established. Dr. Drew was asked to lead this project by serving as the full-time medical director

Dr. Drew did not discover plasma transfusion. In fact the procedure was first proposed and established during World War I. However, Dr Charles Drew established uniform procedures for collecting and processing blood and establishing mobile blood collection units. This work enabled Britain to develop a large scale blood banking project such that there no longer was a need for the United States to supply the British with plasma.

However, Dr. Drew's job was not done. As America grew closer to participating in the War there was a need to establish a plasma collection system for the United States military. Dr. Drew took additional leave away from Howard to lead this project. Without any scientific basis, the military stipulated that blood should only be collected from whites. Shortly there after, Dr. Drew returned to Howard to complete is primary goal of training African American physicians to become outstanding surgeons.

Upon his return, Dr. Drew took and passed the oral exam for certification by the American Board of Surgery. A short while later he was appointed to assume the duties as professor and head of the Department of Surgery at Howard, and became Chief Surgeon of Freedmen's Hospital. For the next ten years Dr. Drew trained half of all the African American surgeons certified by the American Board of Surgery (eight) and many others received part of their training under the direction of Dr. Drew.

Though Dr. Drew is very well known for

See **Drew** next page

Drew: Cont. from previous page

his involvement in the blood banking project, the circumstances surrounding his death, though often erroneous, have made the Drew name famous. On Saturday April 1, 1950 Dr. Drew and three of this colleagues were on there way to Tuskegee, Alabama to attend an annual clinic. Along the way, Dr. Drew fell asleep at the wheel. The car was involved in a severe accident. When the accident subsided, Dr. Drew was the only individual who was severely injured. Dr. Drew and some of the other passengers were rushed to Alamance General Hospital in Burlington, North Carolina. Popular rumor explained that Dr. Drew eventually passed away because the hospital would not admit him or provide him with plasma because he was African-American.

However, as corroborated by physicians at the hospital, the other physician passengers involved in the accident, and Dr. Drew's wife, Minnie Lenore Drew, Dr. Drew was provided with the best possible medical care at the hospital.[8] Dr. Charles Drew did not survive the accident because his injuries were too severe.

Dr. Charles Richard Drew's death at the youthful age of 49 was a significant loss to the entire medical establishment and the African American Community. Though he was consumed by his formal duties and obligations, he found time to volunteer on the boards of numerous professional and public groups.[9] For his achievements with the blood banking project, Dr. Drew has been given many awards and honors. However, those close to him believe that the one aspect of his life that he would never want to be forgotten is his commitment and effort to produce African American surgeons who are at the forefront of the medical establishment.[10] And, For this and all of his efforts he will always be remembered.

Hispanic Women Physicians: Dedicated to the Health of Women & the Hispanic Community

Helen Rodriguez-Trias was born in New York City in 1929. She spent her early years in Puerto Rico. At age 10 she returned with her family to New York City. Helen returned to Puerto Rico to attend the University of Puerto Rico and graduated in 1957.

She enrolled at the University of Puerto Rico School Of Medicine and graduated in 1960 with high honors. She stayed in Puerto Rico and performed her medical residency. During that time, she established the island's first hospital center focused on the care of newborn babies. This effort led to a 50% decrease in the hospital's infant mortality rate.

In 1970, she returned to New York City where she worked in pediatrics and community medicine at Lincoln Hospital, which served a predominantly Puerto Rican section of the South Bronx. In addition, she was also appointed associate professor of medicine at Albert Einstein College of Medicine, Yeshiva University.

Dr. Rodriguez-Trias was an active proponent of women's health. She strove to stop sterilization abuse among poor women of color. She formed the Committee for Abortion Rights and Against Sterilization Abuse and

See **Dr. Rodriguez** next page

Dr. Rodriguez: Cont. from previous page

testified before the Department of Health, Education, and Welfare for passage of the federal sterilization guidelines in 1979. These guidelines require that woman give written consent to sterilization. In addition, the procedure is explained to each woman in understandable language. After the consent is signed, a women is given a waiting period before the procedure can be performed.

After that, she worked on behalf of women with HIV in New York State as the medical director of the State Department of Health AIDS Institute. Dr. Rodriguez-Trias was very active in the American Public Health Association, she helped form its Hispanic Caucus, and later became its first Latina president.

For her tireless work, Dr. Rodriguez-Trias was awarded the Presidential Citizen's Medal for her work on behalf of women, children, people with HIV and AIDS, and the poor. She died in December 2001, around the age of 72.

Sylvia M Ramos was born in Puerto Rico in 1946. However, she grew up in the South Bronx of New York City. Sylvia developed a strong love for science and a desire to help people. She was drawn to medicine as it would allow her to fulfill this desire and provide the least career restrictions. She graduated from the Albert Einstein College of Medicine in 1974. She obtained her general surgical training at Montefiore Medical Center in New York City.

Once she completed her hospital training, she joined the department of surgery as an associate professor. In the department, she was responsible for patient care, medical student and resident education, and directed the surgical nutrition program. She also headed the medical school's office of Special Educational Programs whose focus was to increase the number of underrepresented minority students in medical school.

In 1990, Dr. Ramos left New York City for Albuquerque, New Mexico where she opened her own office. Other career interests include health policy for Hispanic populations and public speaking about breast cancer.

Nereida Correa was born in Puerto Rico in 1946. At age 5 she moved to the Upper West Side of New York City. When she entered high school, Nereida was convinced that she wanted to become a physician. However, her guidance counselors would not support her desire believing that she was not strong enough for medicine and encouraged a career in nursing.

After graduating from high school, she took the counselor's advice and earned an associate degree in nursing from Bronx Community College. She graduated in 1966 at the age of nineteen. For the next fifteen years, she worked as a nurse and helped implement many community programs to support the training of nurses. However, that was not enough and she earned a bachelors and masters degree in nursing education. She then become an assistant professor in maternal-child health nursing for Medgar Evers College. She conducted research and wrote papers on the health and cultural practices among Hispanics and developed courses in nursing leadership and cultural diversity.

The passion for medicine resurfaced as she worked with physicians at Kings County Hospital. She enrolled at Queens College for her pre-medical studies. She finally received

See **Dr. Correa** next page

Dr. Correa: Cont. from previous page

the support and encouragement she needed. Dr. Nereida was accepted to three medical schools, and matriculated to Albert Einstein College of Medicine. She graduated with distinction in psychopharmacology. She then went on to receive residency training in family medicine and obstetrics and gynecology.

In 2002, Dr. Nereida Correa became the first Hispanic woman Chair of the Department of Obstetric and Gynecology at Lincoln Medical and Mental Health Center. She also became a faculty member at the Albert Einstein College of Medicine in the Ob-gyn and Family Medicine departments. Among all her duties, she is most proud of her ability to provide direct patient care, perform surgery, deliver babies, and serve as an advocate for the health and education of women of color. As Chief of the Ob-Gyn department, Dr. Correa enjoys her ability to teach cultural and linguistic competency and influence the standard of care patients receive.

Dr. Percy Julian: A Great African-American Scientist

Percy Julian was born on April 11, 1899 in Montgomery, Alabama. He attended DePauw University where he earned a B.A. degree and graduated in 1920 as a Phi Beta Kappa member and the highest-ranking student in his class. Following graduation, he went to Fisk University where he taught from 1920 to 1922. He then was offered the Austin Fellowship to study at Harvard University in the biophysics and organic chemistry departments. He earned a M.S. degree in only one year. From 1926 to 1927, he served as Professor of Chemistry at West Virginia State College. The following year, he moved to Washington, D.C. and became Associate Professor of chemistry and head of the chemistry department at Howard University. During his time at Howard, he earned his Ph.D. degree from the University of Vienna, in Austria.

Dr. Julian is best known for his achievements in the chemistry lab. He synthesized products that previously only could be found in nature. For example, he synthesized the sex hormones testosterone and progesterone which were used to provide treatment for some forms of cancer and pregnancy disorders. His work with the synthesis of the hormone cortisone led to a less costly manufacturing process enabling it to become more widely available. His work with the soybean led to discoveries in the manufacture of additional drugs, hormones, vitamins, paint and paper products. All his research led to over 100 patents.

Dr. Julian was able to use his knowledge and skill as an entrepreneur. He founded and served as president of Julian Laboratories, inc. and Laboratories Julian de Mexico.

Over the course of Dr. Julian's life he received 19 honorary degrees, 18 academic and civic citations including the NAACP's prestigious Springarn Medal Award, and on January 29, 1993 the United States Post Office honored him with his picture on a stamp.

Dr. Julian died on April 19, 1975 at the age of 76.

Chapter X

Going To Medical School

O nce a student has selected their medical school, they should begin to consider what costs they may face traveling to and getting settled in the city in which the school is located. When looking for apartments, realize that not only do landlords require payment of the first month's rent, but most also require a security deposit which is usually an additional month's rent. To live in the apartment a student may also have to buy furniture and kitchen appliances and pay for phone and utilities service. If a car was purchased consider the cost of auto insurance and if neighborhood parking is limited a student may have to pay for a parking space. Students may also have to pay a parking fee in order to secure a space close to school. In addition, medical schools require a student to have health insurance. Students who are no longer covered under their parent's health insurance plan or are currently uninsured, will be required to pay for the health insurance plan the school offers.

Medical students are expected to have certain equipment when school begins. Some medical schools have a program which enable a student to rent this equipment while other's do not. Contact the medical school about what services they provide. If the school does not have a rental program, be aware that some of this equipment can be very expensive. To reduce this expense, look for used equipment. Upon arriving at school, look for notices on bulletin boards or try checking the medical school bookstore. Waiting too long will reduce the chance of getting a used piece of equipment that is in good condition and conveniently priced.

Another cost of medical school is books. Like college, medical textbooks are very expensive. One method of reducing the first year textbook expense is to save textbooks from the pre-medical classes. For some material covered during your first year in medical school, the only textbooks you may need are the ones you used during your undergraduate career. At the beginning of the school year, many 3rd and 4th year medical students post notices on bulletin boards about textbooks they have for sale. The cheapest books in the best condition go fast so it is wise to look for notices posted on bulletin boards as soon as you get to school and act quickly.

As I will discuss in the next section, many students do not have parents or close family members to provide money to pay for personal expenses or medical school tuition and fees. As a result most students have to rely on other sources of funding such as scholarships, loans, and federal or state programs. It is important to be aware that money applied for or promised are not always immediately available. As a result, it is imperative that you secure for yourself some money to help you relocate and pay for the initial expenses.

Students who take out loans should be aware that loan checks are sent to the medical school's financial aid office. The financial aid office will notify a student to come in and sign the loan check over to the school. Monies from the loan check are first used to pay any balance on that semester's tuition and fees. Only when the balance is paid will a student receive money for personal use. Thus, a student may not receive any or all of the money until the last loan check has arrived. The money that is left over, after paying the tuition, will be given as a refund check. It normally takes 7 - 10 days for the check to be issued.

In the event a student has a full scholarship by the medical school, a government program, or some outside source, it is wise to take the same precautions and have enough money to help relocate and get set up. Like loan money, scholarship money is not always available when the school year begins. If a student is not able able to meet their financial obligations at the beginning of the school year they should not hesitate to contact the schools financial aid office. Many schools have short-term loan funds available for students caught in such a predicament.

A Physician's Prayer

Sovereign Lord,
grant me the opportunity to be a vessel to do your will.
You are the great Physician and Healer.
Guide my hands, my eyes, my ears, and my mind.
Allow them all to work quickly and clearly.
Watch over each patient that I see.
Heal them as it is in your will.
Cover over my iniquities and give me incite when the course is confusing.
I know that each success is a product of your supreme love and nothing about me.
Maintain in me a humble heart and spirit;
never to be overconfident in my own ability and lose focus on you.
Amen

News Flash!

Medical History Gazette

Vol 1, No 10• The First Source for Medical History •Columbia, S.C.

Drs. Antonia Novello & M. Joycelyn Elders
America's first Women Surgeon Generals

On August 23, 1944, Antonia was born in Fajardo, Puerto Rico as the eldest child of Antonio and Ana Delia Coello. Antonia was born with an abnormally large, malfunctioning colon. This chronic medical condition frequently forced her into the hospital. However, when Antonia was eighteen years old her colon was surgically corrected. Happy to be free of the nagging medical problem, young Antonia understood that there were many people who were not so fortunate as she and dreamed of one day becoming a physician so she could help other people with medical problems as she was helped.

Antonia began to pursue her dream of becoming a physician by entering the University of Puerto Rico as a pre-medical student. Antonia graduated with a bachelor's of science degree in 1975 and the following year matriculated to the University's medical school. Antonia's dream became a reality in 1970 when she graduated from medical school.

Dr. Novello continued her medical education at the University of Michigan where she completed an internship and residency in Pediatrics. Upon completion of the residency, Dr.

See **Novello** next page

A native of Schaal, Arkansas, Joycelyn was the oldest of eight children. Upon reflection Joycelyn recalled never visiting a physician prior to her first year in college. At the age of 15, the United Methodist Church awarded young Joycelyn a scholarship which enabled her to attend Philander Smith College in Little Rock, Arkansas.

Upon graduation at age 18, she entered the United States Army as a first lieutenant and received training as a physical therapist. She attended the University of Arkansas Medical School (UAMS) on the G.I. Bill and graduated in 1960. Following graduation, Dr. Elders was an intern at the University of Minnesota Hospital in Minneapolis and subsequently returned to Little Rock, Arkansas and completed her pediatric residency at the University of Arkansas Medical Center in Little Rock. Upon completion of the residency, Dr. Elders obtained a master of science degree in biochemistry and shortly afterwards, 1976, she joined the faculty at UAMS as a professor of pediatrics. She received board certification as a pediatric endocrinologist in 1978. Based on her studies of growth in children and the treatment of hormone-

See **Elders** next page

Novello: Cont. from previous page

Novello went to Washington, D.C. for a pediatric nephrology fellowship at Georgetown University Hospital. Upon completion of the fellowship, Dr. Novello established her own private practice in Springfield, Virginia. However, she quickly found that direct patient care was not cut out for her as she had explained in a magazine interview, "when the pediatrician cries as much as the parents [of the patient] do, then you know it's time to get out."

Dr. Novello was hired in 1978 as a project officer at the National Institutes of Health. She quickly rose through the ranks of the NIH and by 1986 was named deputy director of the National Institute of Child Health and Human Development; one of the NIH's 26 highest positions..

In the fall of 1989 C. Everett Koop, M.D., announced he was retiring after serving eight years as Surgeon General. The Surgeon Generals post was hotly contested. However, Dr. Novello rose above the crowd and on October 17, 1989 President Bush nominated her to become the Fourteenth Surgeon General of the United States of America. On March 9, 1990, Dr. Novello was officially sworn in. As the fourteenth Surgeon General, Dr. Novello became the first woman, first Hispanic, and first Puerto Rican to hold the post.

As Surgeon General, Dr. Novello was the President's spokesperson on issues concerning public health. The Surgeon General is also responsible for overseeing the 6,400 member commissioned corps of whose officers primarily consists of physicians who staff health centers on Native American reservations, serve areas of the country with a shortage of physicians, and help provide medical services during national emergencies among other duties.

Following the footsteps of Dr. Koop, Dr. Novello was in the public spotlight. She championed such issues as tobacco and alcohol advertising, underage drinking, domestic violence, increasing the nation's vaccination rate, and the plight of HIV infected children. In addition, Dr. Novello brought attention to the lack of health care services and health care coverage in the Hispanic American community.

Elders: Cont. from previous page

related illnesses, she wrote more than 150 medical research articles.

In October of 1987, Dr. Elders was appointed to be the director of the Arkansas Department of Health by then Governor Bill Clinton. As director, Dr. Elders achieved many records in areas of public health concern. The number of early childhood screenings in Arkansas increased from just over 4,000 in 1988 to 45,000 in 1992. The immunization rate for two year olds increased from 34% in 1989 to 60% in 1992. In an effort to combat infant mortality, she worked to increase the number of women receiving early and regular prenatal care, with an increase of 17% in the maternity caseload from 1990 to 1992. Dr. Elders expanded HIV testing and counseling services to include every Arkansas county and more than doubled these services since 1990. She expanded the availability of mammogram testing for women with low incomes. In home services for frail and terminally ill patients, including intermittent to continuous care, were expanded to offer 24-hour, seven day a week care.

With this outstanding work record as well as numerous awards and honorary

See **Elders** next page

Elders: Cont. from previous page

doctorates from such prestigious schools as Yale University and Morehouse College, Dr. Elders was nominated by President Clinton to become the 16th surgeon general in the United States Public Health Service on July 1, 1993. Upon senate confirmation on September 7, Dr. Elders was promoted to the rank of three-star admiral. As the 16th surgeon general, Dr. Elders became the first African American woman to hold the post.

Dr. Elders was responsible for the public health service corps, the public health services offices of population affairs, minority health, women's health, and the President's Council on Physical Fitness and Sports. As a theme guiding Dr. Elders' term she stated, "I want to change the way we think about health by putting prevention first. I want to change the behaviors and attitudes of Americans by promoting programs and policies which will enable each of us to be responsible for our own health. I want to be the voice and the vision of the poor and the powerless. I want to change concern about social problems that affect health into commitment. And I would like to make every child born in America a planned and wanted child."

Black Physicians Make History at NASA

Dr. Mae Jemison is the youngest of three children. She was born in Decatur, Alabama and raised in Chicago, Illinois. At sixteen she attended Stanford University on scholarship where she graduated with a Bachelor of Science degree in Chemical Engineering. She attended Cornell University Medical College and received her medical degree in 1981.

She worked as a general physician in Los Angeles and then spent two and a half years as an Area Peace Corps Medical Officer in Sierra Leone and Liberia in West Africa. She then returned to Los Angeles and resumed her medical practice.

She Joined NASA in 1987. On September 12, 1992, Dr. Jemison made history as a crewmember of the space shuttle Endeavor. This was the first African American woman to go into space.

Dr. Bernard A. Harris, Jr. was born June 26, 1956 in Temple, Texas. He received a doctorate in medicine from Texas Tech University School of Medicine. Following residency at the Mayo Clinic, he completed a fellowship at NASA Ames Research Center in California and he studied musculoskeletal physiology and disuse osteoporosis.

Dr Harris joined NASA Johnson Space Center as a clinical and flight surgeon and became an astronaut in July 1991. He participated in two space flights logging more than 438 hours in space. He is the first African American to walk in space. Dr. Harris left NASA in April 1996.

Dr. Yvonne Darlene Cagle received her medical degree from the University of Washington. The Health Professions Scholarship Program sponsored her training. She was commissioned as an officer in the U.S. Air Force. Then she completed residency training in Family Medicine. From her first tour of duty, she was selected to attend the school of Aerospace Medicine at Brooks Air force Base. She then became certified as a flight surgeon. In 1996, Dr. Cagle was selected by NASA as an astronaut and is qualified for flight assignment as a mission specialist.

In May 2004 **Dr. Robert Satcher**, an orthopedic surgeon, was selected as one of NASA's newest astronauts

Chapter XI

"If you are not a part of the solution
you are a part of the problem."
-Eldrige Cleaver-

Financing a Medical School Education

Medical school is very expensive. Normally, during the course of four years, over $100,000 dollars will be invested in your professional education. With this in mind it is important to think about how you want to finance your medical education. The three main options available are loans, private scholarships, and government "scholarship" programs.

Loans

Loans will be the most available option for financing your medical education. The six major government loan programs are:

Loan Program	Interest Rate
1. Federal Stafford Loan (Subsidized)	Capped at 9%
2. Federal Stafford Loan (Unsubsidized)	Capped at 9%
3. Federal Supplemental Loan for Students (SLS)	Capped at 11%
4. Federal Perkins Loan	5%
5. Primary Care Loan	5%
6. Health Education Assistance Loan (HEAL)	Variable
7. Alternative Loan Program (ALP)	Variable

The first five loan programs have to be repaid in ten years while the HEAL loan is 25 years and the ALP loan is 20 years. While in school, the interest accrued from money borrowed from program numbers **1** and **4** are paid by the government while the rest of the programs leave it up to the student to pay the interest while in school. When you apply for financial aid through your medical school, loan money may be provided through one or more of these programs.

There are a number of private organizations that provide low interest loans. Some of the loan programs are structured so that interest will not accrue as long as a student is in school full time. These programs are preferable because over medical school and residency training the amount of interest that can accrue on a loan can become a significant amount of money. Therefore, the more loans a student can find which does not accrue interest while a full time student, the better. It takes some research to find these loan programs. Contact each medical school to which you apply and ask them to provide their financial aid material. Often a number of private organizational loan programs will be included in the material.

If at some point during the undergraduate education a student decides to to take time off before entering medical school, be aware that loan companies will required payment on their loans. If during the payback period a payment or consecutive payments are missed the loan will go into default.

When someone defaults on a loan, the lender has the right to require immediate payment of the **entire** balance. If the entire loan is paid back the student will no longer be in default. Besides paying the whole loan back at one time, some lending institutions will declare a person to no longer be in default if six consecutive on time payments are made. Whatever option is taken, it is important to know that the default episode will be on the credit record which can hinder approval for future loans. If a payment or multiple payments can not be made, it is imperative that the lender is notified. Many lending institutions are often very willing to work out an alternative plan which may include lowering the monthly payment.

It is impossible to find a financial institution willing to give additional student loans to a student that already is in default, was previously in default, or has a very poor credit history (remember those credity cards). As a result, a student that is accepted into medical school may not be able to attend because they can not secure approval for additional loans. The medical school may recommend a one year deferment to pay off the loan in default and improve the credit score.

Private Scholarships

There are many scholarship books available in bookstores and libraries. Unfortunately, most scholarships do not apply to medical students and often those that do exist have residency requirements. Again, as with the search for private organizational loan programs, it is best to begin at the financial aid office of the medical schools to which you apply. Though there are not that many scholarships available, it is still worth your while to look around. You may just find a fifteen hundred dollar scholarship. If you think about it, it may take you five hours to find and apply for the scholarship. If you get a scholarship of fifteen hundred dollars and it took you five hours of work to secure it you just earned three-hundred dollars per hour.

In your scholarship search, you will find a few for students who have completed their second or third year of medical school. This is to make sure the student does not find medical school too difficult, drop out, and not fulfill the goal of the scholarship program. If you find information on scholarships for years other than the first year of medical school, put the information in a safe place. When the time rolls around you can be first in line to submit an application.

Some publications compiling scholarship information include: "The Black Student's Guide to Scholarships by Barry Beckham", "Directory of Financial Aids for Minorities 1995-97 by Gail Ann Schlachter and R. David Webber", "Minority Financial Aid Directory by Lemuel Berry, Jr.".

In addition, in the cities of Washington, D.C.; Cleveland, Ohio; San Francisco, California; Atlanta, Georgia; and New York City, New York, there is a Foundation center whose sole purpose is to help people and organizations find money. The center is a library that contains almost every loan, scholarship, and grant book that currently is in circulation. You can get more information on their web page at http://fdncenter.org/ or stop by and visit. There is no charge for the use of the library. The addresses are as follows:

79 Fifth Avenue/16th Street New York, NY 10003-3076 Tel: 212-620-4230	312 Sutter Street, Suite 606 San Francisco, CA 94108-4314 415-397-0902
1422 Euclid Avenue, Suite 1600 Cleveland, OH 44115-2001 216-861-1934	1627 K Street, NW, Third Floor Washington, DC 20006-1708 202-331-1400
50 Hurt Plaza, Suite 150 Atlanta, GA 30303-2914 404-880-0094	

Government Programs

National Health Service Corps: Scholarship Program

One of the first programs you may want to consider is the National Health Service Corps (NHSC) Scholarship Program. The NHSC is a highly competitive scholarship program available to medical students truly interested in the primary care specialties (Family Medicine, General Pediatrics, Ob-Gyn, and General Internal Medicine) and is committed to serving part of their career in a health professional shortage area. Students accepted into the program will receive tuition support and a monthly stipend. Each year of financial support is offset by a year of service. The minimum service obligation is two-years.

There are three drawbacks to this program. First, this is a primary care driven program and does not support the training of medical specialists. A participant in the scholarship program is locked into pursuing a primary care specialty. Therefore, if there is any doubt in your career choice do not apply to this program but consider the NHSC loan repayment program. The second drawback to this program is that the tuition reimbursement and stipend is considered taxable income. Once tax is taken out, little money is left for actual living expenses. Therefore, the scholarship recipient is still required to take out thousands of dollars in loans. The last drawback to the scholarship program is that once residency training is completed, the participant will have a limited choice of where to serve the years of commitment. Students will be directed to areas of the country with the highest medical need.

Applications to the program are available during the early spring. Students may be able to obtain an application from their pre-medical office, by calling the NHSC application and awards branch at 1-800-221-9393, or visit online at http://nhsc.bhpr.hrsa.gov/. The application to the program consists of a questionnaire. Students are required to answer twenty-five or thirty questions which are formulated to determine the commitment toward working with underserved populations and in underserved regions of the country. Based on the answers to the questions applicants will receive a score. If the score is high enough, the applicant may be selected for an interview. It is from those candidates who are interviewed that the NHSC Scholarships are given.

National Health Service Corps: Loan Repayment Program

This second major government program is similar to the scholarship program except applicants do not apply until the completion of residency training. Prior to applying to this program, a physician has to begin working for an approved medical center. The NHSC maintains a list of approved medical centers. All centers are located in areas of the country with a significant health care need. After employment has been secured with an approved medical center an application can be submitted to the NHSC for the loan repayment program. Applicants who are accepted into this program are provided with:

- Up to $50,000 for 2 years of service
- Up to $85,000 for 3 consecutive years of service
- Up to $120,000 for 4 consecutive years of service

The benefit of this program is that as of 2005 all loan repayment money is provided tax free. In addition, while the loans are being paid back, participants are receiving a very competitive salary and benefit package. Many participants in this program work side by side with doctors who are doing the same job and are receiving the same salary. However, the participants are having their loans paid back while their colleagues are not.

The advantage of this program compared to the scholarship program is that it does not trap a medical student into a primary care specialty. However, the main drawback is that applicants are not guaranteed participation in the program even if they work in a qualifying medical center. The number of accepted applicants is often limited by restrictions in government funding.

Detailed information can be obtained from the NHSC application and awards branch at 1-800-435-6464 or visit their web site at http://nhsc.bhpr.hrsa.gov/jobs/.

U.S. Health Professions Scholarship Program

This program provides scholarships from the Army, Air Force, and Navy. Selected students enter the military as commissioned officers. While completing medical school, students receive a stipend for ten and one-half months, will have all their tuition paid, and will be reimbursed for books and fees. Recipients are expected to perform a 45-day active duty program each year they receive the scholarship. During active duty, full pay and allowances are provided. Active duty training can be performed in a military health care facility where the student will work with military physicians and other members of the health care team. Scholarship recipients will incur an active duty obligation of one year of service for each year a scholarship is received with a two-year service minimum.

After medical school graduation, students are required to apply for one of the military's first year graduate medical education programs as a resident in a military hospital. It is important to note that at any point during residency training, participants may be called to active duty and begin work immediately where a military conflict may be. Once the conflict or active duty obligation is completed residency training may be completed.

Students seriously considering this scholarship should take some time to decide which branch of the military (Army, Navy, and Air Force) is best suited for them. Each military program has different expectations of its physicians. Look into the duties of a physician in the Air Force compared with the Army, and Navy. Get a good understanding of what each doctor does and where they will be assigned during times of war and peace. Take a look into the type of basic training each branch will expect you to perform and think about how such activity might affect your capabilities as a physician. You can find information about the ARMY program at http://www.goarmy.com/amedd/, for the AIR FORCE at http://www.airforce.com under the careers section go to healthcare careers, and for the navy visit http://www.navy.com/healthcare/physicians.

Applying For Financial Aid

Before a student can be considered for any federal loan programs or medical school scholarships, they have to fill out the proper documents. Medical Schools begin to send out the documents around the end of February or the beginning of March. Due to the large number of students a school interviews, the documentation is normally only sent to students who have been accepted. Thus, it is beneficial for a student to interview early so they will have their acceptances when the financial aid material is distributed. Because finances are often an important factor in a students final decision, if the financial documents are returned to the schools quickly, the financial aid officers will send a preliminary award letter. In this letter the school will provide an estimate of how much money will be given in loans and scholarships if the student matriculates to the school. This gives students a chance to compare the financial support from each of the schools.

If you received financial aid during your undergraduate years, the application process is the same. The information that each school requires can be taken from the income tax return filed by the student and their parents. As a result, it is imperative that tax returns are filed as early as possible. This way there will be no delay in filling out each medical school's financial aid application and receiving a preliminary award.

Often after paying four years of college tuition there is not enough money around for some parents to help with the medical school expenses. If you find yourself in this situation don't panic. It is standard policy at each medical school that if you are accepted you will then be given enough financial aid to attend. As a result of this policy, a student's financial background is not a consideration in the medical school selection process.

Financially Deciding What Medical School to Attend

Finances often are a source of great anxiety. Upon choosing a medical school, the anxiety can only increase because medical school is extremely expensive. Most private medical schools range between $33,000 to $35,000 per year for tuition and fees. Many public medical schools range between $12,000 to $17,000 per year. A students first inclination may be to select the least expensive medical school or the school that offers the most financial aid. It is frightening to consider over $100,000 in loans just from medical school.

Upon visiting each medical school keep asking this question: Is this medical school financially worth it? In answering the question, a student should consider what the medical school will offer. Will it provide the options and programs desired? Does it have adequate support resources? Most importantly, will you be emotionally and spiritually happy at this medical school? If after answering these questions, the least expensive medical school is what actually is best, then go for it. But don't be put off by one of the more expensive schools if it is the one that is just right. Medical school is one of the cases where spending more money may be worth it. After all, the money you spend on medical school, is an investment in yourself and your career.

In planning your future, consider the fact that clinical medicine is one of the most secure professions. There has never been a time when a large number of physicians have been unemployed. In economic recession or boom, people get sick. As well, due to the competitive salary physicians receive, there have been few situations where student loans can not be paid. Actually, most physicians are able to pay their loans while still living quite comfortably.

Financial Management

Innocent and unexperienced, college and medical students often do not consider the long term consequences of financial decisions. And, this can cost more money than is necessary. College and medical school's are expensive. Other than a full scholarship, there is no way around paying tuition, fees, room and board. As loans are utilized to pay these expenses, consider the total cost (the principal and interest) of the commitment.

Take enough time to read the "fine print" of any loan and never rush to sign on the dotted line. Look at the interest rate- is it fixed or variable? If it is variable how often can the rate change? Is there a cap on how high the rate can go? Can you pay off the loan early? When will the first payment will be due? Can loan payments be deferred during residency training? How many years will there be to repay the loan? What happens to the status of the loan if a leave of absence from medical school is taken because of personal, health, or family problems? What happens to the loan if you lose your life? will your family have to pay it? What are the penalties for defalting on loan payments?

When considering loan programs, look for loans that will not accrue interest till after medical school and even better till completion of residency training. Verify with the financial aid officer that all these loans have been exausted before agreeing to take out an immediate interest accruing loan. Interest accruing loans begin to cost the day they are signed into existance. The balance can balloon quickly as the interest is compounded with the principal. For example, a $1,000 loan with 6% interest compounded annually will turn into a $1,504 loan after 7 years. Consider the following: if a monthly loan payment is about $660 but the loan obligation increases from $100,000 to $110,000 due to accrued interest while in medical school and residency, the years of repayment would increase from 24 to 30 years and the total paid interest over those years would increase from about $89,000 to $128,000, a difference of $39,000. A young physician can make better use of this money to purchase a house, buy a vehicle, support a family compared with giving it to a bank.

Therefore, if you take out an immediate interest accruing loan, make every effort to pay the monthly interest. To pay this interest, find a job in a lab, tutor college or medical students, etc. Parents and relatives may not be able or willing to pay your tuition, but might assist with your interest only payments.

If possible, do not depend on private loans to pay your educational expenses. Always secure governement based loans first. Private loans typically do not have terms and conditions that favor the student. As well, they often are not eligible for repayment through government programs such as the NHSC Loan Repayment Program. And, based upon current guidelines you can not consolidate private and government loans.

Lastly, after completing residency training you might consider consolidating your student loans. This is a great way to extend your payment terms and lower your payments. However, be cautious about consolidating with a spouse. If you do, the new consolidated loan will not be eligible for loan repayment through the National Health Service Corps.

Total Debt of the 2004 Under-Represented Minority Graduates

Private Medical Schools

$150,000 +	37%
$100,000 to $149,999	22%
$75,000 - $99,999	12%
$74,999 or less	19%
No Debt	10.2%

Total Debt of the 2004 Under-Represented Minority Graduates

Public Medical Schools

$150,000 +	22%
$100,000 to $149,999	32%
$75,000 - $99,999	16%
$74,999 or less	21.9%
No Debt	9.4%

Medical History Gazette

Vol 1, No 11• The First Source for Medical History •Columbia, S.C.

Special Edition

A Guide to America's Minority Medical Association's

The National Medical Association (NMA)

In 1892, Dr. Miles Vandahurst Lynk proposed the establishment of a national Black medical organization in the first editorial of his Journal The Medical and Surgical Observer (the nations first Black medical journal). Three years later, 1895, the "Cotton States and International Exposition" was held in Atlanta, Georgia. At the exposition, Dr. Lynk called for a meeting of the Black physicians in attendance. Twelve physicians met at the First Congregational Church. The idea of a national association was discussed and by unanimous opinion, the National Medical Association for Colored Physicians, Dentists, and Pharmacists was created. Dr. Robert F. Boyd was selected as the first president; Dr. Lynk, vice-president; Dr. D. L. Martin, secretary; Dr. D.N.C. Scott, treasurer; and Dr. H.R. Butler chairman of the executive board. The organization met for a second time in 1903 and shortened its name to National Medical Association.

In 1909, the association began publication of its own journal. Dr. Charles Roman served as its first editor-in-chief. The journal serves as "a medium for publication of medical articles by Negroes [and] a nationwide intercommunication...upon which Negro physician came to rely." This journal is the oldest medical periodical published continuously by Black Americans.

Today, the NMA continues to promote the collective interest of physicians and patients of African descent. Some goals include working toward parity in medicine, the elimination of health disparities and promotion of optimal health, increasing the representation, preservation and contribution(s) of persons of African descent in medicine. There are national programs on Asthma & Allergies, breastfeeding, environmental health, HIV/AIDS, immunization, lupus, tobacco control, traffic safety, and clinical trials. In 2006, the NMA turned 111 years old.

The National Hispanic Medical Association (NHMA)

The NHMA was established in 1994 by Dr. Elena Rios among others. The first national conference was held in March 1997. The organization represents over 36,000 licensed Hispanic physician in the United States. The Mission is to improve the health of Hispanics

See **NHMA** next page

and other underserved populations by working to expand access to quality health care, increase opportunities in medical education, expand cultural competence, and support research for Latinos.

The Association of American Indian Physicians (AAIP)

Fourteen American Indian physicians in Oklahoma joined in 1971 and created the AAIP. The association is dedicated to pursuing excellence in Native American Health care by promoting education in the medical disciplines, honoring traditional healing practices, and restoring the balance of mind, body, and spirit. Today there are more than 300 members participating in organizational activities. The AAIP sponsors the Native American Youth Program that identifies American Indian high school students who desire a career in the health professions and sends them for a week in Washington, DC for a health careers experience. Pre-medical college students can participate in pre-admission workshops held several times a year at various medical schools across the country. The AAIP also sponsors a mentoring and shadowing program for high school, college, and medical students to gain a first person experience of the medical profession. Lastly, the association provides forums and workshops for students to examine and better understand how they can integrate western and traditional medical / cultural practices.

Interamerican College of Physicians and Surgeons

The ICPS was founded in 1979 to promote cooperation among US Hispanic Physicians and to advance their professional and educational needs. The ICPS works to represent Hispanic physicians in the United States, Puerto Rico, Mexico, the Caribbean, Central and South America, and Spain. The goal of the organization is to improve the health of the Hispanic community, reduce the incidence of preventable diseases, improve educational and leadership opportunities for Hispanic physicians, and encourage Hispanic youth to pursue careers in the healthcare field. For the past 20 years, the ICPS has published MEDICO Interamericano as its official scientific Journal and for the past five years Medico de Familia (Family Doctor) a monthly medical digest for the Hispanic community. The ICPS' commitment to Hispanic Youth is accomplished by supporting a mentoring program that pairs Hispanic high school, college, and medical school students with physician mentors.

The Student National Medical Association (SNMA)

In the late 1950's, members of the National Medical Association began to call for the creation of student chapters of the NMA. In August 1961, the NMA Board of Trustees and the House of Delegates approved a motion to "Authorize the establishment of Student NMA chapters at any medical school where they might be desired either by the NMA or the students concerned." In April 1963, a constitution and by-laws were written and the SNMA was officially formed as a

See **SNMA** next page

student section to the NMA. In 1967, the SNMA severed its ties with the NMA and became an independent organization.

Since its inception, the SNMA has grown into over 160 chapters based at colleges and medical schools in the United States and the Caribbean. Though a majority of members are African American, the membership includes student and medical professionals from all cultural and ethnic groups. The SNMA mission is to support current and future under-represented minority medical students and address the needs of underserved communities. National and local programs include health professional recruitment, teenage sexuality, violence prevention, international health, and health screening and education.

The SNMA supports a yearly national conference for pre-medical and medical students.

The National Network of
Latin American Medical Students (NNLAMS)

The NNLAMS was formed in 1987 and incorporated in 2003. The goal is to unify all Latino medical students, promote the recruitment and retention of Latino students, educate medical students on Latino health issues, act as an advocate for the rights of Latinos in health care, etc. The national headquarters is located at The Duke University School of Medicine. As a supporting member of NNLAMS, **The National Boricua Latino Health Organization** (NBLHO) was formed in 1970 by Latino medical students. It represents health professions students from the northeast region of the United States. There are eleven active medical school chapters. The **Latino Medical Student Association**, also a supporting member of NNLMAS, was founded in 1982. Currently there are 13 chapters located in California, Arizona, and Utah.

The Association of Native American Medical Students (ANAMS)

ANAMS was founded in 1975 as an umbrella organization to represent Native American graduate students in the professions of Dentistry, Veterinary, Optometry, Podiatry, Pharmacy, and Medicine. The goals of the organization are to provide support for Native American students enrolled in health professional schools and work to increase the number of Native American students in professional schools.

Chapter XII

begin quote
"There can be hope only for a society which acts as one big family, and not as many separate ones."

-Anwar Sadat-

Careers in Medicine

After you decide on medicine as your career, the next major consideration will be what field of medicine you find appealing. There are endless possibilities and due to the rapid development of medical technology and new methods of healing, it is likely that when you receive your medical degree, new specialties will be emerging. There is also extensive variety within each medical specialty. The result is that after you have completed your medical residency you will be able to tailor whatever medical specialty you choose so that it will satisfy your personal goals and ambitions.

**Top Medical Specialities as Selected by
Minority Medical Student Graduates - 2004**

1. Internal Medicine Subspeciality
2. Family Medicine
3. Surgery
4. Emergency Medicine
5. Obstetrics and Gynecology
6. Anesthesiology
7. Pediatrics
8. Psychiatry
9. Orthopedic Surgery
10. Internal medicine

The following is a short description of the major medical specialties. Once you tell the world of your plans to become a physician, the first question asked is, "What type of physician do you plan to become?" In addition, it is important to be aware of all the options as you enter medical school. However, do not feel ashamed if you enter medical school undecided. It is common for a student to enter with one specialty in mind and leave with an interest in another.

Primary Care Medicine

Primary care medicine is one of the fastest growing areas in medicine due to the nationally recognized need for physicians who are concerned with keeping the population healthy. Primary care consists of those physicians who diagnose and treat almost 80% of the health problems presented to the health care system. The role of these physicians is to provide continuity of care by overseeing the activities of specialists or any other health care professional involved in the care of a patient. The medical specialties that are included in primary care are: Family Medicine, General Pediatrics, and General Internal Medicine. However sometimes, Obstetrics-Gynecology, Emergency Medicine, Psychiatry, Dermatology and Neurology may be included as well.[1] Currently more and more specialties want to be associated with primary care medicine due to the federal government's interest in restructuring the funding and support of the heath care system to focus on primary care.

Family Medicine

The family physician is trained to give medical care to the entire family regardless of sex, age, race, or type of problem, be it biological, behavioral or social. Thus, the family doctor delivers babies, shares the concerns of young families, examines young athletes, assesses risk factors, treats heart attacks, cares for the elderly, and counsels patients. As a counselor, the family physician allows the patient to describe his or her problems and the feelings that attend them. Such a characteristic tends to make the family physician a humanistic and people-oriented type of person.

The family physician is the patient's first stop for recovery from a health problem. In most instances, it is the last stop. However, in a few situations the family physician will refer the patient to a medical specialist for specific care. In such situations, the family physician does not abandon the patient but continues to be the patient's primary advocate in all health related matters.

Though the primary focus of the family physician is the care of patients, some are intimately involved in clinical and epidemiological research. In addition, family physicians are asked to speak at schools and community groups, sharing information about health promotion, disease prevention, and management of common health problems.

Residency training in family medicine takes three years. Some of the major subspecialties associated with family medicine include: geriatric medicine and sports medicine. For more information contact: American Academy of Family Physicians 11400 Tomahawk Creek Parkway, Leawood, Kansas 66211-2672 or visit their internet site at www.aafp.org.

General Internal Medicine

Internal medicine is a medical specialty concerned with the diagnosis and treatment of disorders involving the internal organ systems of the adult. The internist is a diagnostician who takes a comprehensive history, performs a thorough and complete physical exam, records diagnostic impressions, orders appropriate laboratory and diagnostic tests, evaluates the test results, and then treats the patient. Some internists limit their practice to patients with certain diseases or medical problems in one organ system, such as the heart and blood vessels, kidneys, lungs, digestive system, endocrine glands, or blood.

A typical week in the life of an internist will vary depending on the doctor's individual interests and practice arrangements. In general, a large part of the day is spent in the office, seeing new patients and following up on others to determine the effectiveness of therapy or progression of disease.

Residency training in internal medicine normally takes three years. Training in subspecialties require an additional three to five years of training. Some of the subspecialties associated with internal medicine include: Cardiology, Geriatrics, Hematology, Nephrology, Endocrinology, Rheumatology, Sports Medicine, Gastroenterology, Infectious Disease, Pulmonary Medicine, Critical Care Medicine, Diabetes and Metabolism. For more information, please visit the American College of Physician's web site: http://www.doctorsforadults.com/index.html.

General Pediatrics

Pediatrics is the specialty that requires a comprehensive knowledge of the growth and development of children from gestation through young adulthood. Children differ from adults anatomically, physiologically, immunologically, psychologically, developmentally, and metabolically. Thus, pediatricians understand that children are not miniature adults, but instead are in a constant state of physical, developmental, and emotional change. In the past, pediatricians devoted much of their time toward treating infectious diseases. Now they devote their time to providing preventive health care and managing the special long term needs of chronically ill and disabled children.

Though a pediatrician's primary role is to care for the physical health of children, they can fill other roles. Pediatricians are counselors who help children work through developmental, behavioral, and/or emotional problems. As a teacher, a pediatrician may choose to work in an academic hospital, participate in the instruction of medical students, and engage in exciting research. Most importantly though, pediatricians serve as advocates for children in the hospital, community, state, and the nation.

Residency training in pediatrics takes three years. Some of the major subspecialties associated with pediatrics include: Adolescent medicine, Pediatric cardiology, Pediatric endocrinology, Pediatric neurology, Pediatric nephrology, Pediatric rheumatology, Pediatric sports medicine, Pediatric critical care medicine, Pediatric gastroenterology, and Pediatric infectious disease. For more information contact: American Academy of Pediatrics, 141 Northwest Point Blvd. Elk Grove Village, IL 60007-1098. (847) 434-4000 or visit their web site at www.aap.org and do a search under pediatric career information.

Non-Primary Care Medical Specialties

Academic Medicine

Academic medicine is a unique medical field because it encompasses all of the medical specialties but within a medical school teaching hospital setting. An academic physician's work will involve a combination of patient care, teaching, and research. Teaching may involve time spent in the classroom with medical students, in the hospital with residents, or a combination of both. Most of the research is either laboratory or clinically oriented. The degree of time spent in either of these three areas is generally left up to the physician.

Besides the duties previously described, most medical faculty have some type of administrative and committee responsibility including editing medical journals, serving on peer review groups, and obtaining funding for research projects.

Anesthesiology

The anesthesiologist is a vital member of a surgical team and has critical responsibility for the patient's welfare. In the operating room, the anesthesiologist directs or administers the anesthetic, monitors and maintains the vital functions of heart rate and rhythm, blood pressure, body temperature, and respiration. To prevent any unexpected side effects during an operation, every anesthesiologist makes preoperative rounds to establish essential physician-patient rapport and to evaluate the anesthetic experience of the patient and his or her family. Responsibility for patient care does not end upon departure from the operating room, but rather extends into the recovery room. It is the anesthesiologist who determines when a patient can be discharged safely from the recovery room.

Residency training in anesthesiology takes four years. Some of the subspecialties associated with anesthesiology include: Pediatric anesthesiology, Obstetric anesthesiology, Neurosurgical anesthesiology, Cardiothoracic anesthesiology, Ambulatory anesthesiology, Critical care & pain management. For more information about the field of anesthesiology contact: American Society of Anesthesiologists, Inc., 520 N. Northwest Highway, Park Ridge, IL 60068-2573. (847) 825-5586 or visit their web site at www.asahq.org/ and click on their resident and career information section at the bottom of the home page.

Dermatology

Dermatologists are physicians who have expertise in the diagnosis and treatment of diseases that affect the skin, mouth, hair, and nails. With this background and knowledge, dermatologists are qualified to diagnose and treat the wide variety of dermatologic conditions such as skin cancers, rashes, contact dermatitis, acne, hair loss, and scars. They also have expertise in the care of normal skin and in the prevention of skin diseases and skin cancers. Dermatologists perform many specialized diagnostic procedures including skin biopsy, cytological smears, and cultures. Treatment methods include medications, selected x-ray and ultraviolet light therapy, laser surgery and a range of other dermatologic surgical procedures. A dermatologist can see adults and children.

Training in dermatology includes one year of general medical residency training and three years of clinical dermatology training. For more information about the field of dermatology contact: American Academy of Dermatology, P.O. Box 4014 Schaumburg, IL 60168-4014 or call them at (847) 330-0230. You can locate them on the internet at www.aad.org.

Diagnostic Radiology

The field of radiology encompasses a wide range of activities. The activities include the reading of chest films (for pneumonia, pneumothorax, etc.) and bone films (for fracture, tumor, etc.), angiography (the study of vessels involving the placing of a catheter often distant from the point of entry into the skin), to biopsy (where a needle is placed in the site of interest done under ultrasound or CT guidance). In addition, radiologists participate in the service of mammograms (used to search for tumors in the breast), nuclear radiology, magnetic resonance scanning, gastrointestinal radiology (where contrast is introduced either directly or indirectly into the portion of the GI tract in question), ultrasound, and computerized tomography (CT for short).

The radiologist does not see one specific group of people but rather interacts with everyone from the newborn to the geriatric patient. In addition, the radiologist deals with every organ system and nearly every disease state.

Residency training in radiology takes up to five years to complete. For more information about the field of radiology contact: American College of Radiology, 1891 Preston White Dr., Reston VA 22091. (800) 227-5463 or visit their web site at www.acr.org/.

Emergency Medicine

Emergency medicine, the most recently developed medical specialty, encompasses the immediate decision making and action necessary to stabilize patients in health crises. "Emergency physicians deal with the entire spectrum of acute illness and injury in all age groups. Hands on physical diagnosis and the use of both medical and surgical therapeutic modalities are an integral part of the specialty."[5] Often patients are seen in rapid succession, and thus, the emergency physician's greatest challenge is the nearly limitless variety of patients encountered in clinical practice and providing an immediate response to the patient's needs.

Emergency physicians also must work closely with paramedics. The physician not only directs the care rendered by the paramedic out in the field but also directs the care delivered by a wide variety of health care professionals in the emergency room. Other opportunities in this specialty include research to develop newer and/or improved methods of care, work within the community to train residents in basic emergency care, as well as work on the development of community medical disaster plans. Depending on the hospital's location, emergency physicians may work anywhere from 45 to 60 hours a week. Though the hours are long, the work schedule is fixed in advance. In addition there is rarely a call schedule outside of assigned working hours giving the emergency physician greater freedom during off hours.

Residency training in emergency medicine consists of three years of hospital training and up to five years of additional training for an emergency medicine subspecialty. For more information about the field of emergency medicine contact: American College of Emergency Physicians, 1125 Executive Circle, Irving TX 75038-2522. (800)-798-1822 or (972)-550-0911 or visit their web site at: http://www.acep.org/.

General Surgery

The general surgeon has the specialized knowledge and expertise related to the preoperative, operative, and postoperative management of a patient. They are capable of performing procedures involving the gastrointestinal tract, the abdomen and its contents, the breast, the skin, the head and neck, the blood vessels, and musculoskeletal system. General surgeons also can assist in the treatment of cancer patients and those who suffer major traumatic injuries. Surgeons are often able to utilize innovative technology in the surgery suite. In the hospital, surgeons manage the underlying surgical problem in critically ill patients found in the intensive care, trauma, and burn units. Surgeons are able to schedule most of their surgical procedures. However, they can be called to duty at any time of day or night to provide life-saving surgery.

Training to become a General Surgeon takes five years following the completion of medical school. Some of the surgical subspecialties include: Neurological surgery; Orthopedic surgery; Otolaryngology: Head and Neck surgery; Plastic surgery; and Urology. For more information about the field of general surgery contact: The American College of Surgeons; 633 N. Saint Clair St. Chicago, IL 60611-3211 or by phone at (312) 202-5000. On the internet search http://www.facs.org.

Geriatric Medicine

Geriatrics is a branch of medicine that deals with the problems and diseases of old age and the elderly. This field has developed as a specialized part of internal medicine and family medicine in response to the dramatic increase over the past few decades in the number of elderly people. Many medical schools now have a group of full time geriatricians engaged in patient care, teaching, and research. Every practicing physician, outside of pediatrics, will be caring for increasing numbers of older patients. Future physicians with training in geriatrics will find the care of older persons to be one of the most challenging and gratifying careers in medicine, one that involves diagnosing obscure disease, helping to restore mobility, and helping to maintain independence for the many who are now living longer lives.

For more information about the field of geriatrics contact: American Geriatrics Society, The Empire State Building; 350 Fifth Avenue, Suite 801 New York, NY 10118; Phone - 212/308-1414 or visit their web site at: http://www.americangeriatrics.org/.

Obstetrics-Gynecology

Obstetrics involves the care of women before, during, and immediately after the birth of a child. The general obstetrician must be knowledgeable about family planning, endocrinology, infertility, high-risk pregnancy, teenage pregnancy, genetics, as well as surgical obstetrics.

Although babies have been born the same way for centuries, every obstetrician knows that it is likely they will encounter unusual situations during pregnancy, labor, and delivery. The "unusual" is part of the excitement of the field, whether it's the birth of quintuplets in a mother previously treated for infertility or the sudden and potentially disastrous occurrence of hypotension and shock from an inverted uterus just after delivery.

The practice of Gynecology includes the diagnosis, treatment, and prevention of diseases and abnormal conditions of the female reproductive system throughout a woman's life. Most gynecologists treat all age groups, but some physicians are especially interested and qualified in the field of pediatric and adolescent gynecology.

Residency training in Ob-Gyn takes four years. Some of the subspecialties in Ob-Gyn include: Critical Care Medicine, Gynecologic Oncology, Maternal and Fetal Medicine, Reproductive Endocrinology. For more information contact: American College of Obstetricians and Gynecologists, 409 12th Street, SW, Washington, DC 20090-6920; (800) 673-8444 or visit their web site at: http://www.acog.org/.

Ophthalmology

An ophthalmologist is a physician who performs surgery on and cares for all medical conditions relating to the eye. The patient who consults an ophthalmologist is often self-referred or referred by friend or acquaintances. Like other primary care specialists, the ophthalmologist may treat entire families, and is able to provide continuity of care through a patient's entire lifetime.

Most Ophthalmologists practice a combination of medicine and surgery. General ophthalmology ranges from lens prescription, to medical treatment for ocular inflammation, injury or infection, and even to some of the most delicate and precise surgical procedures. In a typical week, the average ophthalmologist may examine more than 100 patients in the office and perform approximately two major surgical operations.

Training consists of one year of general medical training and then three additional years in an Ophthalmology residency program. Some subspecialties in Ophthalmology include: Cornea and External Disease, Glaucoma, Vitreoretinal Diseases, Ophthalmic Plastic Surgery, Pediatric Ophthalmology, Neuro-ophthalmology, and Ophthalmic Pathology. For more information about the field of Ophthalmology, contact: American Academy of Ophthalmology, 655 Beach St. PO Box 7424, San Francisco, CA 94120-7424. (415) 561-8500 or visit their web site at http://www.aao.org/.

Orthopedics

The modern orthopedist specializes in treating disorders of the musculoskeletal system. This includes bones, joints, muscles, tendons, ligaments, nerves, skin, and related structures. Some of these disorders require surgery for correction, others require casting or bracing, and still others may require working with physical therapists, psychologists, and other members of the health care team for rehabilitation. Orthopedists see people of all ages, from newborns with clubfeet, to young athletes requiring arthroscopic surgery, to the elderly needing treatment of arthritis.

Orthopedists spend more time in the office than other surgical specialists do. This allows a high level of patient contact and, in some areas of practice such as rehabilitation and arthritis, long term patient follow-up. The orthopedist's day is generally a busy one, with the average orthopedist seeing a median of 110 patients a week and doing about 20 surgical procedures a month.

Residency training in orthopedics takes five years with an additional one to three years of training for the orthopedic subspecialties of plastic and hand surgery. For more information about the field of orthopedics contact: American Academy of Orthopedic Surgeons, 6300 N. River Road, Rosemont, IL 60018-4262. (847) 823-7186 or visit their web site at: http://www.aaos.org/.

Physical Medicine and Rehabilitation

Physicians in this specialty are called physiatrists (fizz ee at' trists). They care for patients with acute and chronic pain, and musculoskeletal problems like back and neck pain, tendonitis, pinched nerves and fibromyalgia. They also treat people who have experienced catastrophic events resulting in paraplegia, quadriplegia, or traumatic brain injury; and individuals who have had strokes, orthopedic injuries, or neurologic disorders such as multiple sclerosis, and polio. They see patients in all age groups and treat problems involving all the major systems in the body. These specialists focus on restoring function to people.

To become a physiatrist, students must successfully complete four years of medical school and four additional years of residency training. Residency training includes one year spent developing fundamental clinical skills and three additional years of training in the full scope of the specialty. Many physiatrists choose to pursue additional advanced degrees (MS, PhD) or complete fellowship training in a specific area of the specialty. Fellowships are available for specialized study in such areas as musculoskeletal rehabilitation, pediatrics, traumatic brain injury, spinal cord injury, and sports medicine.

To obtain additional information about this specialty contact the American Academy of Physical Medicine and Rehabilitation at One IBM Plaza, Suite 2500 Chicago, IL 60611-3604 or call at (312) 464-9700. On the web search under: http://www.aapmr.org/.

Psychiatry

Psychiatry is a medical specialty devoted to mental, emotional, and behavioral conditions. It deals with many illnesses in which the source of the symptoms is obscure, from both biological and psychogenic aspects. A psychiatrist seeks to obtain information about past events that were emotionally meaningful to the patient, and to examine his or her usual way of reacting to people and events. The psychiatrist attempts to construct an emotional profile by this examination. Once a relationship between psychological reactions and symptoms is established, a plan of treatment is developed. Such treatment may take place in an outpatient facility or a hospital.

Residency training in psychiatry takes up to four years. Some of the subspecialties associated with psychiatry include: Clinical neurophysiology, Addiction psychiatry, Child & adolescent psychiatry, and Forensic psychiatry. For more information about the field of psychiatry contact: American Psychiatric Association 1000 Wilson Boulevard, Suite 1825, Arlington, Va. 22209-3901 or visit their web site at: http://www.psych.org/.

Other Careers in Medicine

As described in this chapter's introduction, the beauty of being in the field of medicine is that there is a world of opportunity for everyone. The above career fields are just a small snapshot of the available opportunities. Physicians can get involved in state or federal government as elected officials and become leaders in evaluating and writing health policy or work for health organizations as government lobbyists. As well, physicians are the leaders within the Department of Health and Human Services, The Centers for Disease Control and Prevention, The Surgeon Generals Office, and the National Institutes of Health. Physicians are leaders in advocacy organizations such as the American Cancer Society and American Heart Association. Physicians are involved in bringing health to the world through the World Health Organization and various Church sponsored mission projects. Physicians are leaders of the business world via managed care organizations, health care networks, and hospital administration. Lately, it has become common for popular magazines to have physician writers who regularly contribute information on healthy living. As well, physicians are becoming involved in broadcast journalism and work for local and national television stations / networks serving as medical correspondents.

For additional information on the various medical specialties, I suggest you visit the Association of American Medical Colleges' web site at (http://www.aamc.org/students/cim/) and explore their "careers in medicine" page.

News Flash!

Medical History Gazette

Vol 1, No 12• The First Source for Medical History •Columbia, S.C.

Dr. Satcher Appointed by President to lead the CDC:
Becomes its first African American Director

David Satcher was born in Anniston, Alabama on March 2, 1941. He was one of eight children raised on a farm in rural Alabama. At the age of 2, David contracted a severe form of whooping cough and his parents were told by the only Black physician in the area that he would not live through the illness.[1] However, great motherly care enable David to survive and continue a life full of promise.

For many young African American boys and girls growing up in the south at this time in American history the many dreams never flourished into reality. However, this would not be the case for David's dream of becoming a physician. Though David's parent's formal education ended in elementary school, they understood the value of an education and required all eight of their children to attend school even though the family farm could have used their help in the fields.[2]

At the peak of the civil rights movement, David left Anniston for Atlanta, Georgia where he attended Morehouse, College. At Morehouse, David excelled in his classes and was honored by being elected to the Phi Beta Kappa scholastic fraternity. David continued his education at

In 1982, Dr. Satcher was selected as the eighth president of Meharry Medical College. From 1993 to 1998 he was director of the CDC and from 1998 to 2002 served as U.S. Surgeon General.

Case Western Reserve University School of Medicine, Cleveland, Ohio. At Case, he earned a M.D. degree, a Ph. D. for his research in cytogenetics, and was elected to the Alpha Omega Alpha Honor Medical Society. Dr. Satcher completed his medical training at Strong Memorial Hospital, Rochester, New York.

Dr. Satcher's career began on the west coast where he served as associate professor in community medicine and director of the community outreach hypertension program at the Charles R. Drew Postgraduate Medical School in Los Angles. A few years later, Dr. Satcher developed and served as chairman of the Department of Family Medicine and also became Dean of the Drew Medical School. As Dean, Dr. Satcher worked toward integrating the work of his school to meet the needs of the surrounding community. For these efforts he received the Watts Grassroots Award for Community Leadership. In 1979, Dr. Satcher moved to Atlanta, Georgia where he served for three years as Chairman of the Department of Community Medicine and Family

See **Satcher** next page

Satcher: Cont. from previous page

Practice at Morehouse College of Medicine.

In 1982 David Satcher, M.D. was selected to become the eighth president of Meharry Medical College Nashville, Tennessee. As one of three historically Black Medical Schools, Meharry has been in existence for 122 years and has trained over 40% of the nations African American Physicians. As President, Dr. Satcher faced an ominous predicament. The city's White-controlled Metropolitan Nashville General Hospital was aging and in need of a new building. Meharry's affiliated medical center, Hubbard Hospital, needed to establish a larger patient population. Dr. Satcher concluded that the solution would be to merge the two medical centers with Meharry taking charge of patient care and administrative duties. "Fear about entrusting medical care to Black doctors and administrators" swept through the minds of many people in the White medical community.[3] However, after four long years of negotiations, the merger was formalized.

On November 15, 1993 the Secretary for the Department of Health and Human Services, Donna E. Shalala, announced that David Satcher, M.D. was appointed by President Clinton, to be the Director of the Centers for Disease Control and Prevention (CDC) and Administrator of the Agency for Toxic Substances and Disease Registry (ATSDR). As the first African American director of the CDC, Dr. Satcher was in charge of the primary governmental agency responsible for promoting health and preventing disease, injury, and premature death. The CDC employs over 7,000 people in Atlanta and across the nation and has an annual budget of over $2.5 billion dollars. At the announcement ceremony Dr. Shalala stated, "Dr. Satcher brings world-class professional stature, management skill, integrity, and preventive health care experience to his job".

From the CDC, Dr. Satcher was appointed by President Clinton to become the 16th Surgeon General. Following confirmation by the United States Congress Dr. Satcher was sworn in on February 13, 1998. Dr. Satcher continued his drive to educate the nation on such health concerns like violence, AIDS, poor immunization rates, and alcohol abuse. Though some of these issues were new to America, many had been a part of American's minority community for decades.

In 2002, Dr. Satcher became director of the National Center for Primary Care at the Morehouse School of Medicine. The Center's mission is to promote excellence in community oriented primary care and optimize health outcomes with a special focus on underserved populations and the elimination of health

An Address by the President of the United States

On August 14, 1968, the President of the United States, the Honorable Lyndon B. Johnson, addressed the National Medical Association at the organizations 73'rd annual convention in Houston, Texas. This became the first time that the sitting President of the United States had ever elected to address a national convention of physicians. In the address, President Johnson focused on issues such as jobs, health, education, housing, medicare, and the movement toward a society free of discrimination.

disparities

Chapter XIII

What If I Am Not Accepted Into Medical School?

This is the dreaded event for every aspiring pre-medical student. In 2004, only 49.4% of all applicants to medical school received an acceptance letter. This means that of the 35,735 applicants, 18,073 of those applicants did not receive an acceptance letter and were forced to resolve this question.

In the event that you come face to face with this situation, there is one thing you should know. YOU ARE NOT A FAILURE!!! It is quite acceptable to be angry, depressed, and go through a lot of "if I had just _____ I would have been accepted" as you question what went wrong. In addition, it may be difficult to tell family and friends. However, do not psych yourself out believing you are stupid, unintelligent, or will not amount to anything. These are the exact beliefs about people of color the dominant culture has been trying to perpetuate for the past couple hundred years. Unfortunately, people of color are still trying to fight this perpetuated myth.

It may take some time to get over the shock. However, one needs to think about the future. There are two main options available for a student in this predicament. Work on applying to medical school again or establish a new exciting career option.

Applying to Medical School a Second Time Around

Applying to medical school again is not easy and requires hard work. Every year there are applicants who reapply to medical school. Many are accepted and become very successful physicians. Students who are not accepted into medical school often did not perform well in their pre-medical courses, on the MCAT exam, or with the application / interview. To find out your areas of weakness call the admissions office of the schools you applied and ask their opinion. If your grade point average was too low ask how you can improve your academic standing. If there were one or two key classes, you may need to retake them. If it was the MCAT exam, retake it. If you interviewed poorly, practice your interview technique. If you chose to apply to the most competitive medical schools, you will need to re-apply with a diverse portfolio of schools. Consider applying to more in-state schools especially if you applied to more out-of-state schools that normally accept few out-of-state students. If your recommendations were poor or just average, work to get better references. If you submitted your application late in the interview season, submit it again in a timely fashion.

Applying Once is Enough

If you decide to end the pursuit of medical school do not despair; there are an enormous number of options and opportunities available to you. Though the task ahead may seem impossible, remember: you made it this far, through enormous hurdles and obstacles. Now the only thing that can stop you is yourself.

When you reflect on your pre-medical career, did you find that you dreaded the pre-medical classes? That may have been the reason you did not perform as well as you liked. It is hard to do well in an area that is not stimulating to one's soul. What courses did you excel in and/or found the most stimulating. Maybe you should consider a career relating to one of those areas. A quick pit stop in your school's career placement office is a great place to start.

However, if you are you still excited about working in the health care field, the health care field needs you. If you love the patient interaction and the value of helping people, then consider becoming an advanced nurse practictioner, physician assistant, physical or occupational therapist, or pharmacist. Other career opportunities include becoming a medical artist and illustrator, health educator, dietitian, nutritionist, health statistician, computer programmer, music therapist, corrective therapist, school health educator, recreation therapist, health sociologist, public health educator, public health program director, social worker, medical science researcher, medical technologist, psychologist, counselor, hospital administrator. Minorities are needed in all of these fields. Whatever choice you make, will be a good choice for the community.

Medical History Gazette

Vol 1, No 13• The First Source for Medical History •Columbia, S.C.

News Flash!

Neurosurgeons Break Barriers and Set Major Achievements

Dr. Alexa Canady: First African American Woman Neurosurgeon

On November 7, 1950 Alexa Irene Canady was born in Lansing, Michigan. The Canady family lived outside the city of Lansing Michigan where Alexa and her brother attended elementary school. Alexa writes of this experience, "My brother and I were the only Black students in the local elementary school. During the second grade I did so well on the California reading test that the teacher thought it was inappropriate for me to have done that well. She lied about what scores were mine and, ultimately, she was fired."[1] Alexa continued to excel in school and graduated high school as a National Achievement Scholar.

Alexa attended college at the University of Michigan and received a Bachelor's of Science degree in 1971. She continued her education at the University of Michigan School of Medicine and graduated as a distinguished member of the Alpha Omega Alpha Honorary Medical Society. Dr. Canady left Michigan for a one year internship at Yale New Haven Hospital and

See **Canady** next page

Dr. Ben Carson Directs Team that Separates Twins Joined at the Head

On September 18, 1951 one of the world's greatest future pediatric neurosurgeons was born in Detroit, Michigan. When Ben was eight years old his parents divorced and he and his brother, Curtis, lived with their mother, Sonya Carson.

Ben's first revelation of becoming a doctor occurred at age eight after joining the Seventh Day Adventist Church. He was inspired by story after story of missionary doctors who were able to relieve physical suffering and help people live happier and healthier lives.

By the time Ben reached the fifth grade, the prospect of becoming a physician looked slim. He was academically last in his class and remarked, "I missed almost every question on just about every test, but when the whole class - at least it seemed like every one there - laughed at my stupidity, I wanted to drop to the floor." However, a short while later Ben received a new pair of glasses and remarked, "I could actually see the writing on

See **Carson** next page

Canady: Cont. from previous page

then was chosen to become a resident in the neurosurgery department at the University of Minnesota. Dr. Canady writes of her opportunity, "When I got a residency in neurosurgery, I got it not because I'm smarter than somebody forty years ago, but because the politics were such that they needed a Black woman and I was there and qualified."[2] Upon completion of the residency program Dr. Canady became the first African American woman to become a neurosurgeon, in the United States.

Dr. Canady continued her education with a fellowship in pediatric neurosurgery at Children's Hospital in Philadelphia, Pennsylvania. Upon completion of the fellowship, Dr. Canady returned to Michigan and joined the Neurosurgery department of Henry Ford Hospital. Later, she became head of the pediatric neurosurgery department at Children's Hospital of Michigan. In 1984 Dr. Canady earned her Board certification from the American Board of Neurological Surgery.

Carson: Cont. from previous page

the chalkboard from the back of the classroom". From that time on, Ben rose to the top of his class and with the help of his mother, his ultimate cheerleader,- "Bennie, you can do it. Don't you stop believing that for a second." - Ben graduated from high school at the top of his class.

Ben chose to attend college at Yale University on a scholarship and went on to study medicine at the University of Michigan. In medical school Ben discovered neurosurgery and fell in love with it. After graduating from medical school, Dr. Carson went to Baltimore's Johns Hopkins Hospital to perform his internship in general surgery. Upon completion of the internship, Dr. Carson was accepted into the hospitals neurosurgery residency program becoming the first-ever African American in the program.

At the end of the residency, Dr. Carson and his family moved to Australia where he was able to perform numerous surgeries and fine tune his skills. Dr. Carson and his family came back to the United States about a year later, and Dr. Carson was hired at Johns Hopkins Hospital as a surgeon. A year later Dr. Carson was promoted to direct the pediatric neurosurgery department; he was thirty-four.

As a pediatric neurosurgeon, Dr. Carson was often called upon to perform delicate procedures such as hemispherectomies in which a portion of the brain is removed to restore a seizure victim to normal functioning. Dr. Carson's most famous operation came in 1987 when he directed a team of 70 doctors, nurses, and medical personnel to aid in the separation of a pair of West German Siamese twins who were joined at the back of their heads. Preparation for the operation took five months and the operation itself consumed almost 22 hours. The historic surgery was successful and two viable healthy young children were produced when only one child usually survived a separation procedure.

Though Dr. Carson has risen to the top of his profession he has not forgotten those following his footsteps. Dr. Carson often creates time to travel and visit students in all parts of the country.

References

Chapter I.

Imhotep: The World's First Great Physician

1. Some ethical precepts of the ancient Egyptian physician are very much like the Hippocratic Oath in sentiment and expression, and this alone would suggest that pre-Hippocratic medicine in Greece owed much to Egyptian medicine.

   Garrison, H. Fielding, History of Medicine W.B. Saunders Co. 1927, 57.

2. "Iu-em-hetep" means "he who cometh in peace". This name was translated to the Greek language as "Imouthes" and the in modern times became "Imhotep".

   Finch, Charles S. The African Background to Medical Science. (London, Karnak House, 1990) p.80.

3. Finch, Charles S. p. 75-76.
4. Egyptians employed cursive script usually etched upon thin sheets of the papyrus leaf.
5. Garrison, H. Fielding. P. 55.
6. Green, John R. Medical History for Students. (Charles C. Thomas, Springfield, Illinois, 1968) p. 17.
7. Garrison, H. Fielding. P. 54.
8. Green, John R. P. 17.
9. Green, John R. P. 14-15.
10. The Caduceus is a symbol used to identify the medical field. It is composed of a staff with two wings on the top and two serpents (snakes) winding up the shaft.
11. --------------- "Origin of the Caduceus Motif." Journal of the American Medical Association 202 (Nov. 13, 1967) P. 615-619.

Medicine in the New World

1. Francisco Flores, History of medicine in Mexico via http://www.somosprimos.com/heritage.htm
2. Nancy Neff, MD "Folk Medicine in Hispanics in the Southwestern United States" Department of Community Medicine, Baylor College of Medicine. http://www.rice.edu/projects/HispanicHealth/Courses/mod7/mod7.html
3. Julia Rombough "Aztec Medicine" http://lark.cc.ku.edu/lance/Family/Julia/HIScover.htm
4. "Native American Medicine" WholeHealthMD.Com http://www.wholehealthmd.com
5. Victoria Abreo "Native American Healing" BellaOnline: The Voice of Women http://www.bellaonline.com
6. Marbella, Anne M. et al. "Use of Native American Healers Among Native American Patients in an Urban Native American Health Center". Archives of Family Medicine 91988;7) 182-185.

Chapter II:

1. AAMC: Minorities in Medical Education: Facts and Figures 2005.
2. American Association of Medical Colleges. Report on Minority Students in Medical Education: Facts and Figures 2004.
3. AAMC Data Warehouse: Applicant Matriculant file as of 2/28/2003.
4. City College of New York Program in Premedical Studies: A student's handbook.
5. John R. Thornborough, Hilary J. Schmidt. The Successful Medical Student Achieving Your Full Potential. (ILOC, Inc. New York, 1993) 74-75.

The Top 10 Colleges Producing Minority Medical School Applicants

1. AAMC: Minorities in Medical Education: Facts and Figures 2005. Pages 77-81.

African Americans in Medicine the Journey Begins

1. Morais, Herbert M. The History of The Negro in Medicine. (New York: Publishers Company Inc., 1967) 12-13.
2. Bousfield, M.O. "An Account of Physicians of Color in the United States." Bulletin of the History of Medicine. Vol. XVII (January 1945) 63.
3. Genovese, Eugene D. Roll Jordan Roll: The World the Slaves Made. (New York: Vintage Books, 1976) 225.
4. Cobb, W. Montague, MD, Ph.D. "The Black American in Medicine." Journal of the National Medical Association. Vol.73 Supplement (1981): 1199.
5. "Blacks in Medicine." The Ebony Handbook. (Chicago: Johnson Publishing Company Inc.: 1974) 361.
6. Wilson, Donald E., MD. "Minorities and the Medical Profession: A Historical Perspective and Analysis of Current and Future Trends" Journal of the National Medical Association Vol. 78 (1986) 177.

Chapter III:

Profile of 2004 applicants to medical school

1. AAMC: Minorities in Medical Education: Facts and Figures 2005. Pages 80-83

Dr. James McCune Smith Fights a War of Words Against Senator Calhoun

1. Morais, Herbert M. The History of the Negro in Medicine (1970, Publishers Company, Inc. New York) 32, 212-213.
2. ----------------. "James McCune Smith." Journal of the National Medical Association 44 (March 1952): 160.

Black Physicians Refuse Push to Go Back to Africa

1. "Blacks in Medicine." The Ebony Handbook. (Chicago: Johnson Publishing Company Inc.: 1974) 361.
2. Delany, Martin Robison. The Condition, Elevation, Emigration, and Destiny of the Colored People of the United States Politically Considered. (New York: Arno Press, 1968) 135.
3. Bousfield, M.O. "An Account of Physicians of Color in the United States." Bulletin of the History of Medicine. Vol. XVII (January 1945) 66.

Dr. John Sweat Rock Speaks out against Slavery

1. Contee, Clarence G. "John Sweat Rock, M.D., Esq., 1825-1866." Journal of the National Medical Association Vol. 63 (May 1976) 237-242.

Chapter IV:

1. Kenneth V. Iserson, M.D. Getting Into A Residency. (Arizona: Galen, 1993) 271.

African American Women Break the Color Barrier in Medicine

1. Aptheker, Bettina. "Quest for Dignity: Black Women in the Professions, 1865-1900." From Black Women in American History: From Colonial Times Through the Nineteenth Century. Darlene Clark Hine ed. (New York: Carlson Publishing Inc., 1990) 97
2. Darlene, Clark Hine, ed. Black Women in America: An Historical Encyclopedia. (Carlson Publishing Brooklyn: 1993) 290-291, 401-402, 682, 387-388.
3. Toyomi Igus, ed. Book of Black Heroes: Great Black Women in the Struggle. (Just Us Books, Inc. 1991) 88.
4. Seraile, William. "Susan McKinney Steward: New York State's First African-American Woman Physician". From Black Women in American History: From Colonial Times Through the Nineteenth Century. Darlene Clark Hine ed. (Brooklyn, New York: Carlson Publishing Inc., 1990) 1217-1234.
5. Cazort, Ralph J. "Susan McKinney Steward (1847-1918) Physician, Hospital Founder, Women's Rights Activit." From Smith, Jessie Carney ed. Notable Black American Women. (Detroit: Gale Research Inc., 1992) 1077-1079.

Chapter V:

1. AAMC: Data Warehouse: Applicant Matriculant File as of 11 / 6 / 2003.
2. Under-represented Minority include: African American, American Indian, Mexican American, Mainland Puerto Rican, C'wealth Puerto Rican, and Hispanic.

**Drs. Susan La Flesche Picotte & Lillie Rosa Minoka Hill Become
America's First Native American Women Physicians**

1. "Dr. Susan La Flesche Picotte." NIH: Changing The Face of Medicine.
   http://www.nlm.nih.gov/changingthefaceofmedicine/physicians/biography_253.html
2. "Dr. Lillie Rosa Minoka-Hill." NIH: Changing The Face of Medicine.
   http://www.nlm.nih.gov/changingthefaceofmedicine/physicians/biography_226.html

Dr. Daniel Hale Williams Performs Historic Heart Surgery

1. Cobb, W. Montegue. "Daniel Hale Williams." Journal of The National Medical Association Vol. 45
   September 1953.

Drs. Williams and Mossell Open Nations First Black Run Hospitals

1. Mossell, M.F. "The Modern Hospital Largely Educational." Journal of the National Medical
   Association Vol. 8 (July-September 1916) 134.
2. Bousfield, M.O. "An Account of Physicians of Color in the United States." Bulletin of the History
   of Medicine. Vol. XVII (January 1945) 66-67.

Chapter VI: Successfully Choosing a Medical School

1. Association of American Medical Colleges: Minority Students in Medical Education: Facts and
   Figures vii. 66
2. AAMC Data Warehouse. March 25, 2002.

Top Allopathic Medical Schools - Table

1. AAMC "Minorities in medical Education: Facts and Figures 2005. 98-102

**Dr. Barnes Becomes First Black Physician Admitted to American
Board of Otolaryngology**

1. Cobb, W. Montague. "William Harry Barnes." Journal of the National Medical Association Vol 47
   January 1955 p. 64 - 66.

Demand for Black Physicians Promotes the Establishment of Black Medical Schools

1. Morais, Herbert M. The History of the Negro in Medicine. (New York: Publishers Company Inc.,
   1967) 40-48
2. Cobb, W. Montague, MD, Ph.D. "The Black American in Medicine." Journal of the National
   Medical Association. Vol 73 Supplement (1981) 1218-1219.
3. Cobb, W. Montague, MD, Ph.D. "Henry Fitzbutler." Journal of the National Medical Association.
   Vol. 44 (September 1952) 403-407.

4. Savitt, Todd L. "Entering A White Profession: Black Physicians in the New South, 1880-1920." Bulletin of the History of Medicine. Vol. 64 (Winter 1987) 512.

Chapter VII: Medical School Application

Ohiyesa (Charles Eastman) An American Indian Physician

1. "Massacre At Wounded Knee, 1890," EyeWitness to History, www.eyewitnesstohistory.com (1998).
2. "Dr. Charles A. Eastman Ohiyesa (Winner) Wahpeton Dakota." www.kstrom.net/isk/stories/authors/eastman.html (1996).
3. "Ohiyesa (Charles Eastman) World Wisdom books, www.worldwisdom.com/author/ohiyesa.asp.
4. David Reed Miller "Eastman, Charles (Ohiyesa)" Encyclopedia of North American Indians http://college.hmco.com/history/readerscomp/naind/html/na_010800_eastmancharl.htm

Dr. Numa P. G. Adams Becomes First African American to be Named Dean of a US Medical School

1. Cobb, W. Montague M.D. "Numa P.G. Adams, M.D." Journal of The National Medical Association Vol. 43 January 1951 p 43 - 52.

Chapter VIII: Medical School Admissions

Dr. Hector P. Garcia: A Fight to Break Down Barriers

1. "Justice for my people: The Dr. Hector P. Garcia Story. http://www.justiceformypeople.org

Chapter IX: Financially Surviving the Medical School Application Process

Dr. Charles R. Drew leads the way in Blood Banking Project

1. Cobb, W. Montague. "Charles Richard Drew, M.D., 1904-1950." Journal of the National Medical Association Vol. 42 July 1950 p. 238 - 246.
2. Craft, Patrick P. "Charles Drew: Dispelling the Myth." Southern Medical Journal Vol 85 December 1992 p.1236 -1240.

Hispanic Women Physicians: Dedicated to the Health of Women & the Hispanic Community

1. "Dr. Helen Rodriguez-Trias" NIH: Changing The Face of Medicine. http://www.nlm.nih.gov/changingthefaceofmedicine/physicians/biography_273.html
2. "Dr. Sylvia M. Ramos" NIH: Changing The Face of Medicine. http://www.nlm.nih.gov/changingthefaceofmedicine/physicians/biography_258.html

3. "Dr. Nereida Correa" NIH: Changing The Face of Medicine.
   http://www.nlm.nih.gov/changingthefaceofmedicine/physicians/biography_70.html

   Dr. Percy Julian: A Great American Scientist
1. http://kato.theramp.net/julian/bio.html

Chapter X: Going to Medical School

**Dr. Antonia Novello Sworn in as Surgeon General: Becomes
First Woman and Hispanic to Hold Post.**
1. Graham, Judith, ed. Current Biography Yearbook 1992. New York: The H.W. Wilson Company, 1992.
2. Telgen, Diane and Jim Kamp, eds. Notable Hispanic American Women. Washington, D.C.: Gale Research Inc., 1993.

**Dr. M. Joycelyn Elders Sworn in as America's 16th Surgeon General:
Becomes first African American Woman to Hold Post**
1. Elders, M. Joycelyn. Curriculum Vitale. U.S. Public Health Service, Department of Health and Human Services.

Black Physicians Make History at NASA
1. All NASA biographies obtained from the NASA web site: www.nasa.gov

Chapter XI: Financing a Medical School Education

Total Debt Table
1. AAMC: Minorities in Medical Education: Facts and Figures 2005. page 103

National Hispanic Medical Association
1. www.nhmamd.org

National Medical Association
1. Summerville, James. "Foundation of a Black Medical Profession in Tennessee, 1880 - 1920." Journal of the Tennessee Medical Association. Vol. 76 (October 1983) 645
2. Cobb, W. Montague, MD, Ph.D. "The Black American in Medicine." Journal of the National Medical Association. Vol. 73 Supplement (1981) 1231.
3. Savitt, Todd L. "Entering a White Profession: Black Physicians in the New South, 1880-1920." Bulletin of the History of Medicine. Vol. 64 (Winter 1987) 638-639.

4. Hansen, Axel C. "Black Americans in Medicine." Journal of the National Medical Association Vol. 76 (1984) 694.
5. Cobb, W. Montague. "The Pursuit of Excellence Project Arcturus." Journal of the National Medical Association Vol. 83 (2) 109.
6. Cobb, W. Montague. "Integration in Medicine: A National Need." Journal of the National Medical Association Vol. 49 (January 1957) 4.
7. Morais, Herbert M. The History of The Negro in Medicine. (New York: Publishers Company Inc., 1967) 68.
8. Cobb, W. Montauge. "Robert Fulton Boyd." Journal of the National Medical Association. Vol 45 (May 1953) 233-234.

The Association of American Indian Physicians

1. http://www.aaip.com/

Inter-merican College of Physicians and Surgeons

1. http://www.icps.org/main.htm

Student National Medical Association

1. www.snma.org
2. "The Need for a Student Auxiliary to the N.M.A." Journal of the National Medical Association Vol. 53 (July 1961) 406.
3. "The Student National Medical Association." Journal of the National Medical Association Vol. 55 (May 1963) 240.
4. "Student N.M.A. Chapters." Journal of the National Medical Association Vol. 53 (November 1961) 659.
5. Mitchell, Oscar. "The Student National Medical Association: A First Message." Journal of the National Medical Association Vol. 57 (May 1965) 250-251.

The National Network of Latin American Medical Students

1. www.nnlams.com

The Association of Native American Medical Students

1. http://www.aaip.com

Chapter XII: Careers in Medicine

1. Kenneth V. Iserson, MD. Getting into a Residency: A Guide for Medical Students. (Tucson" Galen Press, 1993) 8, 23.
2. Doris Gorka Bartuska, MD, "Career Choices for Women in Medicine" American Medical Women's Association. 2 (1984): 6.
3. Kathryn E. McGoldrick, MD, FACA "Career Choices for Women in Medicine" American Medical Women's Association 1 (1984): 2.
4. Charlotte H. Kerr, MD "Career Choices for Women in Medicine" American Medical Women's Association 1 (1984): 15.
5. Nancy E.R. Webb, MD "Career Choices for Women in Medicine" American Medical Women's Association 1 (1984): 18.
6. Nancy Nichols, MD "Career Choices for Women in Medicine" American Medical Women's Association 1 (1984): 13.

Top Medical Specialties as Selected by Minority Medical Students - 2004
1. AAMC: Minorities in Medical Education: Facts and Figures 2005. 104

Dr. Satcher Appointed by President to lead CDC: Becomes first African American Director
1. Applebome, Peter. "C.D.C.'s New Chief Worries as Much About Bullets as About Bacteria." The New York Times 26 Sept. 1993: Sect. 4 p. 7.
2. "CDC head David Satcher receives Board of Trustees Service Award." Case Western Reserve University Medical Bulletin Spring 1995: p. iii.
3. "Introducing: David Satcher, M.D.." Ebony January 1994 pp. 80 - 82.
4. United States Department of Health and Human Services. "David Satcher (1998-2002)." http://www.surgeongeneral.gov/library/history/biosatcher.htm

An Address by the President of the United States
1. Johnson, Lyndon b. "An Address to the National Medical Association." Journal of the National Medical Association Vol. 60 (November 1968) 449-454.

Chapter XIII: What if I am not Accepted into Medical School?

Dr. Alexa Canady: First African American Woman Neurosurgeon
1. Lanker, Brian. I Dream A World. New York, Stewart, Tabori, & Chang: 1989 P. 128.

2. Smith, Jessie Carney ed. Notable Black American Women. Detroit; Gale Research Inc: 1992 P.155-156.
3. LaBlanc, Michael L. ed. Contemporary Black Biography: Profiles from the International Black Community Volume I. Detroit; Gale Research Inc. 1992. P.48-49.

Dr. Ben Carson Directs Team that Separates Twins Joined at the Head
1. Carson, M.D., Ben with Cecil Murphy. Gifted Hands: The Ben Carson Story. New York: Harper Paperbacks 1990.

Appendix

A. Sample Resume
B. The Pre-Medical College Student Timetable
C. Hispanic-Serving Health Professions Schools
D. Hispanic Centers of Excellence
E. Native American Centers of Excellence
F. 10 Sample Essays for the AMCAS Application
G. Questions to Ask During the Medical School Interview
H. Sample Interview Questions for Applicants
I. Resource Information

Sample Résumé

School Address
Street
City, State, Zip code
Phone Number

Permanent Address
Street
City, State, Zip code
Phone Number

PROFESSIONAL SUMMARY

I plan to pursue a career in medicine in association with my interests in Primary care Medicine and Public Health. I specifically am interested in addressing medical problems through social and behavioral changes. I have a wide variety of leadership and organizational skills which I plan to utilize as a primary care physician.

EDUCATION

Brown University - Providence, Rhode Island   Expected Date of Graduation: May 1993
      B.A.- Comparative Study of Development.

University of Ibadan - Ibadan, Nigeria   Summer 1992
      University of Pennsylvania & University of Ibadan links Programme
      Courses taken: 19th and 20th Century African History and African Folklore

Emory School of Public Health - Atlanta, Georgia   Summer 1991
      Course taken: Health Issues in Minority Populations
      Project: James W. Alley Training Program - Health Promotion Resource Center

EXPERIENCE

            Morehouse School of Medicine-Health Promotion Resource Center, Atlanta, Ga.
Public Health Summer Fellowship   Summer 1991
      * I took the results from five different Georgia county health coalition's health needs assessment survey and independently created and constructed for each county coalition a 30 page data analysis-summary of the survey results. The data was presented using computer generated charts and graphs. Besides the final results of the survey population's health status, the charts and graphs included state and national data to allow each coalition the opportunity to better assess the health of their community. Major additional duties included library research and data analysis.

Wright State University School of Medicine, Fairborn, Oh.

Horizons in Medicine Summer Research Fellowship Summer 1989

    Department of Pharmacology and Toxicology
- *Researched the reaction of smooth muscle cells to cytosolic free magnesium using spectrofluroscopy.
- *Lab organizer and carried out experiments on a flurospectrometer
- *Input Data into computer and plotted experimental results

Horizons in Medicine Summer Fellowship Summer 1988
- *Worked with patients in the physical therapy department at the Ohio Masonic elderly Home in Springfield, Ohio

HUMAN RELATIONS

Brown University Development Office-Brown University Spring 1993
- * Office Assistant

Green Memorial Hospital- Xenia, Ohio Summer 1990
- * Worked in the Housekeeping Department.

Brown Student Security - Brown University 1990 - 1993
- * Dispatcher and Shuttle - Escort driver

HONORS / AWARDS

-Emory University, Morehouse School of Medicine, Centers for Disease Control, Public Health Summer Fellowship

-Public Health Summer Fellowship: Award for Outstanding contributions to the program.

-Two year recipient of the Springfield Area alliance of Black School Educators Award for Scholastic Achievement.

PROFESSIONAL ASSOCIATIONS / VOLUNTARY ACTIVITIES

Brown University Soccer Player (89)

Brown University Winter Minority Recruiter (89/91)

Brown University Orientations and Welcoming Committee - Event Organizer. (90 & 91)

African Sun- Historical Events writer for the Black student newsletter (91/92)

Committee on University Reform (CURe) - Writer, Researcher, Section coordinator of a landmark 150 page report on University Minority Affairs. (91/92)

Students On Financial Aid - Publicity coordinator, Treasurer, Event organizer (90/93)

TRAVEL EXPERIENCE

Liberia, Kenya, India, Ethiopia, Bahamas, Spain, France, England, Nigeria

The Premedical College Student Timetable

Year	Sept	Oct	Nov	Dec	Jan	Feb	March	Apr	May	June	July	Aug
1	Organize your pre-medical classes so you can take the MCAT exam the spring of your Junior (3rd) year.		Talk with upper classman at your school and ask about their premedical experience to give you an idea of what to expect ahead.		Following winter break begin looking for medical oriented summer programs or research opportunities. Remember that most programs ask for recommendations.	Be prepared and watch for dealines.				Enjoy Your Summer		
2	Decided on a Major Yet? Thinking about traveling abroad in your Junior year? Don't be afraid to revise your pre-medical academic program but be sure to keep your eye on the prize: **Medical School.**				Begin investigating summer programs in an area of interest. Watch the bulletin board and visit your pre-medical office regularly to see if new announcements have arrived.		Save your textbooks from your pre-medical courses; they are valuable for MCAT review and medical school use.		Be prepared and watch for dealines.	**Have a Good Summer**		
3	If you plan to take the spring MCAT exam give yourself a light academic load in the spring so you will have time to study and prepare.		Over winterbreak decide how you want to review for the MCAT exam. (April) — Don't forget about summer; look for exciting programs available to you.				Time to take the MCAT exam! (April) — Ask your professors to write you a letter of recommendation for medical school. March - April.		What medical school are you applying to? Research the AMCAS / AACOMAS application. Be prepared to fill it out when the application season begins.	**Have a Good Summer**		
4	Time to fill out your secondary applications and send them in.		Time for Interviews and Acceptances				Last month to decide on which allopathic medical school you want to attend without losing your deposit. (May)		**Happy graduation. You earned it!**	Have you made plans for the summer? Don't be afraid to take some time and relax. Have Fun! You need to be mentally prepared when medical school begins.		

Hispanic-Serving Health Professions Schools (HSHPS)

http://www.hshps.com/index.html

Albert Einstein College of Medicine – Yeshiva University (Bronx, NY)
Baylor College of Medicine (Houston)
Charles R. Drew University of Medicine and Science (Los Angeles)
Columbia University College of Physicians and Surgeons (New York City)
Cornell University Weill Medical College (New York City)
Dartmouth Medical School (Hanover, NH)
Harvard University Medical School (Boston)
Nova Southeastern University, College of Osteopathic Medicine (Fort Lauderdale, FL)
Stanford University School of Medicine (Stanford)
Texas Tech University Health Sciences Center at El Paso School of Medicine
The University of Arizona, College of Medicine (Tucson)
University of Washington School of Medicine (Seattle)
University of California Davis School of Medicine (Sacramento)
University of California Los Angeles, David Geffen School of Medicine (Los Angeles)
University of California San Diego, School of Medicine (La Jolla)
University of California San Francisco, School of Medicine
University of New Mexico School of medicine (Albuquerque)
University of Texas Health Science Center at San Antonio Medical School (San Antonio)
University of Texas Medical Branch at Galveston
University of Kansas School of Medicine (Kansas City)
University of Illinois at Chicago College of Medicine
University of Miami School of Medicine
University of Medicine & Dentistry of New Jersey – New Jersey Medical School (Newark)

Hispanic Centers of Excellence
http://bhpr.hrsa.gov/diversity/coe/default.htm

Baylor College of Medicine (Houston)
Stanford University School of Medicine (Palo Alto, Ca)
University of Arizona College of Medicine (Tucson)
University of California – San Diego School of Medicine
University of California – San Francisco School of Medicine
University of Illinois at Chicago
University of Medicine & Dentistry of New Jersey (Newark)
University of North Carolina – Chapel Hill
University of Puerto Rico Medical Science Campus School of Med. (San Juan, PR)
University of Texas at Galveston Medical Branch
University of Texas Health Science Center – San Antonio

Native American Centers of Excellence
http://bhpr.hrsa.gov/diversity/coe/default.htm

University of Minnesota Medical School at Duluth
University of Oklahoma Health Sciences Center College of Medicine (Oklahoma City)
University of Washington School of Medicine (Seattle)

10 Sample Essays
for the AMCAS Application

Sample Essay #1

About one year ago I watched a young African American male, age 25, die in a homicide. I heard two gunshots and ran to the scene to give my assistance. No one would go near him as he lay in the field of grass adjacent to my home. Screams of sorrow and dismay pierced my ears as I knelt over his paralyzed body. The blood and matter ran down the side of his face from the bullet wound in his right temple. He also had a wound in the abdomen. As I checked his fading pulse, his eyes stared into the dark blue skies as if he had already gone. The paramedics arrived soon thereafter, announced him D.O.A., but he was not dead when I arrived: he was very much alive.

I have always said I wanted to be a doctor, someone who could save lives, but I never knew how much I wanted to be a doctor until that night. The guilt that I felt, not having the knowledge or tools to save him, made me realize that my desire to aid people through the medical field is real.

As a member of an ethnic group currently under-represented in medicine, it is my desire to focus on a community that is similar socially, economically, and politically to the community from which I was raised. I grew up in a socio economically deprived development called "The Hough Area" in the city of Cleveland, Ohio. I have a deep emotional attachment to my community because this environment was the fuel to my drive in obtaining a challenging education, one that could lead me back and prepare me to be a servant and role model to the future successors of this deprived but dynamic community. It has always been a dream of mine to create a clinical environment with positive patient-doctor relationships. It is from this that trust and commitment from the people in my community will evolve. With trust and commitment comes a positive attitude about preventive health care. It is my opinion that my community needs more medical practitioners from within, to explain the importance of consistent preventive health care for every member of the family. I am someone who has come from their background, experienced the same problems, understands their situations, and can look at the emotional, social, and physical state with a relative understanding. Therefore, it is my desire as well as my duty to act on my opinion. We must stop the cycle of recurrent but preventive illnesses from generation to generation by educating our children on how to take care of themselves; a health promotion campaign. My decision to pursue a medical career is firmly rooted in the needs of the community of which I am a product and a member.

Sample Essay #2

As a Black woman growing up in America, my experiences and observations of the injustices and persecutions suffered by racial minorities and the underclass are integral to my decision to become a doctor. This flame of injustice and persecution is being fed by ignorance, fear, and mis-education. These in turn contribute to the poor health and minimal or inadequate health care received by the underclass. My decision to become a doctor is based on my strong desire to be able to actively make a difference. I want to contribute as much as I can to society in order to help rectify the aforementioned problems.

Whether it be in classes or away from the classroom, I believe involvement is the best way to learn and master what it takes for the application of skills and problem solving abilities that the medical profession requires. Taking courses gives me the basic knowledge I need but not the "hands-on" experience. Realizing this spurred me to seek an independent study in research work. This involvement in research led to a greater understanding of much of what I had been learning in classes. My first experience was exposure to the technical aspects of molecular biology laboratory work. I learned procedures and techniques that involved electroelution, fusion protein induction, dialysis, sonication, and the use of an SDS page gel. These procedures and techniques proved very useful after I was awarded a summer internship by the Signal Transduction Training Group at Iowa State University. This was a competitive program funded by the National Science Foundation. My summer project has now been extended to an independent study this year. The present project involves using in-situ hybridization to map a gene in order to determine its locus. While doing research, I have discovered that things do not automatically happen as they are explained in books. Although this can be frustrating, the autonomy granted me by my mentors allows me to learn how to think through situations when things are not going smoothly. This has helped enhance my thought process, problem solving skill, and perseverance.

Another one of my goals is to try to educate all those I can reach in order to get rid of the ignorance, fear, and mis-education that is at the root of all social and racial inequality. I tried to accomplish this by being involved in events and organizations that stress leadership and foster multiculturalism and diversity. This is illustrated by the extra curricular activity and jobs I have been involved in. In a competitive interview process that evaluates leadership, management, and personable skill, I was chosen to be resident assistant. As a resident assistant, my job is not just to "police" rules and regulation. It ranges from answering trivial questions to dealing with situations that can be potentially life threatening. Through such experience, I have also had to learn how to keep performing in times of great stress that can be caused by trying to be a counselor for 60 women. Building a community of acceptance and understanding from a floor of 60 strangers is another task I try to tackle as a resident assistant.

College has been a great learning experience for me in all aspects of life. I have made mistakes and I have tried to learn from all of them. In my noble quest to try to eradicate all society's ills, I over-committed and over-extended myself. This caused my performance in some classes to suffer. After some self-evaluation, I realized I needed to observe my limitations and abide by them. Although I strongly feel the need for involvement in activities that make a difference, I also recognize the importance of fulfilling academic requirements according to the best of my abilities. Therefore, I have focused more on class work and tried to balance this with my involvements in other activities. This has been reflected in a much improved grade point average, which I feel is more indicative of my academic ability.

Although I am now trying to do what I can to help society, I know I could contribute most to society by pursuing a medical degree, and if possible, a masters in public health as well. If given this opportunity, I plan to do whatever I can to help cure the diseases plaguing our society as well as the people in it.

Sample Essay #3

My interest in medicine evolved from an interest in engineering. In high school I wanted to be a biomedical engineer. So the summer after my junior year in high school I participated in a summer research program in engineering at the University of Michigan. The research I participated in that summer gave me firsthand exposure to the fields of science, engineering, and, almost accidentally, the field of medicine.

The laboratory in which I worked was located in the heart of the University of Michigan's teaching hospital, around the corner from the Intensive Care Unit. The research project required that electrocardiograms be collected daily from patients in the ICU. As many days as my work allowed, I would throw on my lab coat and join the medical student who would take the EKGs. Those afternoons gave me an opportunity to see the student interact with patients and doctors. It also gave me a chance to talk to her about her experiences in medical school, and to my delight, place a few recording leads on a willing patient.

Since that rewarding summer I have been working towards becoming a physician. I admire the rapport physicians have with their patients and the appreciation patients have for their physicians. I eagerly look forward to the challenge of making a difference in the lives of my patients.

Realizing the demands of a medical training, I have sought ways to enhance my skills to become a successful medical school applicant. I have spent the past two summers performing research at the University of Pennsylvania. The first summer I helped design a protocol for a proposed clinical study of pharyngitis caused by group c beta-hemolytic streptococci. The following summer I analyzed statistical data for an evaluation study of the institution's Geriatric Education Center. The program not only sharpened my experiences in research, but it has also given me valuable clinical exposure in the emergency room and to the fields of internal medicine, sports medicine, gynecology, geriatrics, and even acupuncture. During these clinicals I have often spoke one on one with patients about their lives and medical histories.

The various leadership positions I have held in college have given me tremendous insight in working with people and acting responsibly. As the President of the Health Career Club I was constantly in communication with my peers, faculty, and community physicians in order to orchestrate the many activities of the organization. After running track for two years I became the team captain in my junior year; however, when my injuries became too severe for me to continue running competitively, I decided to relinquish my position on the team and return as the hurdle coach. I hated leaving the team, but through the whole experience I realized that the two years I spent as a collegiate hurdler taught me how to cope with tremendous physical and mental stress as well as to assess my priorities.

Through my experience as an undergraduate I have learned that physicians are dedicated individuals who come from varied backgrounds and are greatly challenged in diagnosing and treating their patients. I am confident that I possess these qualities and am positive that there is a place for me in medicine as a physician.

Sample Essay #4

My interest in medicine and my commitment to that career goal evolved from three important people in my life; my mother, my oldest sister, and my daughter. My mother, originally from Jamaica, has been a registered nurse for more than 25 years. As early as my preschool years, I can recall watching my mother ready herself for work. I would constantly question her, " Mommy, what do nurses do?" She would reply, "We take care of sick people and help them get better." Being impressed with her persona and the idea of helping people get well, I concluded that I wanted to be just like my mother, I wanted to be a nurse. My mother experienced nursing as a career where she was limited to following doctors' orders. She had been placed in situations where her valuable information was disregarded because of her position. Therefore she advised me not to settle for being a nurse but to strive for the best, become a doctor. Though I do not subscribe to the same philosophy of nursing, I do believe that for me, becoming a doctor is becoming the best. My mother planted the seed of interest in me.

My sister encouraged my initial interest and nurtured it into my goal of becoming a physician. Six years after my sister came to the U.S. from Jamaica she was diagnosed as being sickle-cell anemic. At the time, she was 13 and I was 7 years old. The disease did not manifest itself until she was in high school, during which time, she experienced crises of varying severity. Being very close to my sister, I hated to see her in pain. When she experienced a crises I would take her temperature, call the doctor, give her pain medication, apply warm compresses and accompany her to the emergency room. Knowing of my interest in medicine, my sister would always say, " hurry up and become a doctor so I can be your first patient." At that point, I wanted to find a cure or better treatment for sickle-cell. Though my interest in hematology and research has diminished, my sister still has volunteered to be my first patient regardless of which specialty I choose.

My daughter, Ashley, has been a constant motivational force in fueling my commitment to my goals in medicine. Throughout high school I worked diligently to maintain an excellent academic record while participating in many extracurricular activities. In 1988, at the age of 17, I found that I was expecting a baby. My strength and determination were put to the test. I thought my dreams were crushed, my parents thought that I had given up and everyone watched and waited for my life to crumble. With God, my family, my close friends, determination, and self-motivation I completed high school with honors and was accepted to Case Western Reserve University.

In retrospect, I realized that there was no alternative. Ashley deserves the best mother I am capable of being. For me to be the best mother for Ashley, I must first be the best that I can be. Being the best that I can be means fulfilling my dreams of becoming a physician. No child needs the guilt of knowing that her mother's dreams were aborted due to her arrival in her mother's life. I am not saying that my educational endeavors have been easy for either of us. Finding and maintaining the delicate balance between motherhood, academics, work, and the social aspects of my life has been my most difficult challenge. As I approach graduation, I feel comfortable saying that I have found ways for harmonizing motherhood with the responsibilities that accompany the traditional academic pursuits.

My past experience have equipped me with the skills, techniques and incentives to be successful in any challenging situation, including a rigorous medical school program.

Sample Essay #5

As a young boy growing up in Chicago, I was surrounded by a warm family that provided love and support. My family was also initially responsible for sparking my interest in the medical field. Rummaging through my grandfather's medical bag for toys was my first exposure to medicine. My mother saw my eager interest and continued to foster it by providing me with science books. As my curiosity for medicine increased, my mother then encouraged me to spend time and talk with physicians. By taking advantage of those opportunities, I gradually gained more insight into the medical profession.

Of all my experiences, my time volunteering during my college years in the emergency room (ER) of Grady Memorial Hospital (Atlanta, Georgia) was the most insightful and memorable. The experience not only provided clinical exposure, but a chance to affect the lives of others. Assisting physicians and nurses weekly, I observed trauma situations and experienced the emotional and physical demands required of physicians. Transporting patients and delivering lab specimens were my primary responsibilities in the ER. Performing them assured me that my auxiliary support was necessary for the ER's efficiency. The highlight of my experiences came through talking with a diversity of patients. Although I could not help their medical needs, it was very satisfying to provide emotional support through conversation. Patients responded positively and appreciated that someone spent time with them amid the confusion in the ER. This experience showed me that patients are ordinary people with anxieties, problems, and concerns. Although their physical conditions need to be treated, their emotional needs must be addressed also. I am grateful for the opportunity to have fulfilled patient's needs by working in the ER. This clinical experience coupled with others have convinced me that I can meet the demands of the health profession.

My diverse interaction with other people also helped me in other areas. Having the responsibility of a resident assistant taught me to be firm with handling uneasy situations among my peers. Initially, the job was difficult because many residents were friends. However, I knew I needed to remain assertive to have decorum on my floor. Tutoring first year students taught me the importance of listening. I was better able to provide help each time I carefully listened to my student's problems. Lastly, my recent research experiences at Case Western Reserve University has taught me the importance of teamwork. Communication is essential for a research team to ensure experimental procedures are performing properly. Initially I made many mistakes, but later found my errors made me a responsible and independent thinker.

Preparation for a medical career is time consuming and stressful. However, I have found outlets to fulfill my personal needs. My love for art has allowed me to continue to create the many sketches from my wild imagination. In addition, I have found a new interest in photography and intend to learn more by enrolling in a course this fall. Tennis is also a very strong interest I have acquired while attempting to relieve the stresses of school. Finally, my favorite pastime is listening to music from my extensive library of classical jazz and reggae music.

A young boy's dream of becoming a doctor to save the world from diseases is today becoming a reality. My personal interests, family influences, and clinical experiences have all shaped my decision to pursue a career as a physician. I desire a profession which directly benefits others, constantly challenges my mind, and satisfies me daily. Through investigation, I found that a physician's career provides all of those aspects. In the future, My medical preparation will continue to challenge every part of me. However, in a few years I envision myself gaining personal fulfillment by influencing lives as a practicing physician.

Sample Essay #6

At the very early age I learned about the diversity of people. I was born in Ghana, West Africa. I stayed with my Uncle and his Italian wife at age four while my mother went to Ames, Iowa for graduate study. A year later joined her and my new father. A journey along the West Coast and across the U.S. to Ames is etched in my memory. We moved back to Ghana when I was seven but four years later we returned to the U.S.

Between the ages of seven and eleven, while in Ghana, I would accompany my mother, a nutrition consultant, to a nutrition rehabilitation center. The sight of many sick children, mostly my age but smaller because of severe malnutrition, was saddening. I learned that much of the malnutrition could have been prevented by the mothers if they had adequate knowledge of nutrition. Visiting the clinic sparked a strong interest in health care for me.

My parents have encouraged my interest in health care, but they have also cautioned me that I should not pick a career out of sentimentality, that I should have a real idea of what would be demanded of me. Since childhood, pediatrics has been the area of medicine which interests me the most. The interest grew when I worked in a convalescent home in Columbus, Ohio the summer before entering college. The pediatric ward of the convalescent home gave me the opportunity to learn about the fragile nature of children and also about their resiliency. I was part of an experimental group of aides who were hired to provide additional stimulation to the children. Initially, reading stories to some of the bedridden children was distressing because they did not respond the same way my healthy siblings responded. As I continued to read, joke and play with the children, I found that they could react, perhaps not with the same intensity, but they would react. Working with the families of the children was the greatest eye opener to me. I found that I could make a difference in the way the parents felt by showing that I was sincerely interested in the well being of their children. Working in the convalescent home strengthened my initial desire to work with children.

Other experiences have helped me improve my ability to relate to and collaborate with different groups of individuals. During my first year at Oberlin college I worked with Oberlin town elementary children on Saturdays. This volunteer activity included tutoring some children academically, as well as teaching them about nutrition, exercise, and cultural awareness. I was an active participant in my dorm from my freshman year. In my junior year, I accepted the position of a Resident Coordinator of the dorm. This position involved organizing tasks and collaborating with residents to complete projects. Learning to resolve conflict and respect various view points were the important skills I learned from being in charge of over 35 residents. I have had two research experiences. The first was in the summer of 1988 when I assisted in a project involving the characterization of a protein. The research, which was at the Biochemistry Department of the Ohio State University, resulted in a publication, titled Chemical Modification of Spinach Plastocyanin using 4-chloro-3,5-dinitrobenzoic acid: characterization of four singly modified form. in Biochimica et Biophysica Acta, 1016 (1990) 107-114. The second was in the summer of 1992 at Case Western Reserve University. The studies involved looking for the expression of a proto-oncogene in brain tissue under different respiratory conditions. My participation included assisting in the formulation of the research question and carrying out the experiments.

What I have experienced so far has reinforced my desire to go into the health profession. In all these experiences, I have found myself comfortable in dealing with different age groups, acceptable to authority, willing to learn and consider other peoples viewpoints, and yet able to work independently when necessary. These qualities have helped me learn how to be sensitive and handle people with compassion in different circumstances. I know these traits will be important aids as I continue my preparation to become a physician.

Sample Essay #7

The idea of becoming a doctor first came up in a conversation with my father. It was right before my freshman year of high school and we were talking about what I wanted to do as a career after school. I said that maybe I'd be a kindergarten school teacher, since I like working with children. My father looked at me and said, "Have you ever thought of being a doctor? In fact, you could be a children's doctor." Interesting though that sounded, I quickly dismissed the idea for I'd never been to any doctor that I could remember. Anyway, being a doctor meant causing people pain, or so I thought. That conversation was soon forgotten. Not too long afterwards high school began and with high school came field trips to many different places, one of with was a doctor's office. After talking with him and listening to the sound of heartbeats through his stethoscope, it was like kismet! I'd found my niche in the world! I never did see that doctor again, but in my case, once was all it took. I too was going to be a doctor!!

Years later, I was told by a physician and friend that: "Being a medical doctor is not just about taking care of the sick. You have to like taking care of people. You have to be willing to stop everything at the drop of a hat when that call comes in. Its about being the first one out of the house in the morning and the last one in at night. It is about making physical, mental, and emotional sacrifices for the rest of your life and liking it!! That is what being a medical doctor is all about!"

Upon hearing these words, I had to stop and take stock of things. 1). I'd wanted to be a doctor ever since my second year of high school. 2). Yes I actually like helping people, but sacrifices? What types of sacrifices? Sleep? Well, clinical studies have shown that the human body can function on less than three hours of sleep a night. Food? A muffin, here, a slice of piazza there and I'll be happy. Mental? As long as I have a good book and good music I'll be alert and fine. Emotional? Ahh! I'll be the first to admit that I am saddened by the merest hint of human tragedy. But is that all it takes to disqualify me from being a doctor? I hope not!!

With much enthusiasm I've spend the last few school years in preparation for achieving this goal of being a doctor. My summers have been spent in different cities, in programs geared towards those interested in the health professions. Thus far, I've had three summers of research, two at the University of Minnesota and one at New York University Medical Center. Those three summers, along with the summer spent volunteering at the Children's Hospital in St. Paul, have provided me with exposure to the different areas of the health profession.

Though focused and committed to obtaining this goal, I've been able to pursue other interests as well. Over the past three year at Xavier I've been involved in Mobilization at Xavier (M.A.X.), the volunteer organization on campus for which I've served in the capacity of mentor, big sister, and an elementary in-school-tutor. In addition, I am a member of several other clubs and organizations on campus. Among these are the Biology Club, for which I am president-elect for the upcoming school year; Xavier's Gospel Choir, which provides me with spiritual nourishment; The Peer Dean Staff, for which I served as a group leader; and the Inter-Dormitory Council, of which I'm a founding member. And finally my favorite organization, intramural basketball, for I've come to realize that it is only with both mental and physical exertion that I am my best.

In all honesty, I feel that I was meant to be a doctor. I like working with and for people. Upon the completion of my medical training, I hope to be able to spend a portion of my time, up to three months a year, practicing in a third world country, preferably in my home country of Liberia, West Africa. On a final note, I've been advised by many that this personal statement is a very important part of the application process. In that case I hope that this introduction of myself has sufficiently sparked your interest in my abilities. Given the chance I feel that I will make a caring, compassionate, and good doctor. This however, can only come to be if a strong medical institution believes in me as much as I believe in myself and is willing to give me a chance.

Sample Essay #8

During my high school experience, I completed a self-discovery/career exploration course through the Center for Leadership Development (CLD) in Indianapolis, Indiana which proved valuable to my career choice development. The program aims to expose inner-city youth to career opportunities and to develop their leadership skills. Through CLD, I had the opportunity to observe and to talk with a physician who provided me with a realistic outlook about medicine. I was especially impressed by one statement that he made. "The strenuous demands of being a physician are negated by the satisfaction I feel when a patient smiles because of something I have done to help him or her." This comment reinforced my desire to become a doctor.

My commitment to pursue a medical career was further influenced by my attendance at the "Symposium on Biomedical Careers in Science" sponsored by the National Institute of Health in 1989. At this conference, I was introduced to the many opportunities available in scientific research, medicine, and a combination of the two fields. My interest in science has always been one of the primary motivating factors in my desire to become a physician. For the summer of 1992, I pursued my research interests through an internship with Eli Lilly and Company under the supervision of Dr. Ronald Wolff in the area of inhalation toxicology. The research involved working with rhesus monkeys to determine the effect of anesthesia on the bronchoconstriction caused by methacholine. The aim of the study was to develop the ability to measure pulmonary function in conscious monkeys to later be used in anti-asthma research. The internship allowed me to learn more about the relationship that exists among research, the pharmaceutical industry, and the health care field. The experience was invaluable.

I know that as a physician I would be able to fulfill my desire to be of service to others while also satisfying my interest in science. I look forward to medical school as an opportunity to finally learn the answers to all of the questions that I have about how the body functions and is affected by disease. Medical training would allow me to learn these things and apply them clinically. I also anticipate becoming a doctor because, in my daily life, I encounter many of society's major health concerns through family members or close friends who suffer from them. Such experiences motivate my thirst for medical knowledge so that one day I might be instrumental in preventing such occurrences. After my volunteer experience in the emergency department of Indiana University Hospital, my decision to enter the medical profession was solidified. Everything I observed served to reassure me that my decision to enter the health field was the right one.

I am aware that, in addition to a great sense of dedication, appropriate academic ability is a necessity for successful completion of medical training. I believe that my academic record and accomplishments serve as evidence of my ability to be a successful medical student. Such accomplishments include being salutatorian of my 1989 graduating class, being on the Dean's list and receiving the Distinguished Alumni Service Award among other honors. I honestly believe that my clinical and research exposures, in addition to my academic preparation, have prepared me to meet the demand of medical training. I look forward to medical school matriculation and the journey that follows.

Sample Essay #9

I expect to be challenged by the problems and changes that I encounter in my interactions with humanity, as they relate to the science of medicine. I want to participate in the rigor and dedication that the community of doctors share in order to reach the goals of healing. My experiences in medical research and humanities, and in clinical settings have confirmed my desire to preserve health by first learning and then teaching others.

The first time that I saw life under the microscope, the shining cells magnified the beauty in life visible to the naked eye. The details, which we do not fully understand, entice me to embark on the profession which will offer me the opportunity to continue to learn, throughout life, about life. Through my exciting project at the Pittsburgh Cancer Institute, I learned and used many laboratory techniques which may decipher the pathway of an oncogene that disrupts the differentiation of promylocytes into granulocytes. I see that the scientific values of medical research serves as an applicable foundation for clinicians who are also in problem solving situations daily as they interact directly with patients.

I communicated with many people who had varied opinions of and experience with physician, as I compiled the handbook, Cultural Competency Relevant to Specific Cultural Groups in Cleveland. I observed that by addressing the cultural complexities that frame views of health, life, and death, I will better achieve my goal of healing and preserving life. I learned that all people regardless of backgrounds share the desire to be treated respectfully, in what may be fearful confrontations with medicine. My experience as a residential counselor, leader of organizations, and facilitator or workshops on cultural competency and human relations has demonstrated that effective communication with a broad range of people is necessary. In order to remember the interactions that I have had with friends and counselees who have felt uneasy about the problem that they are facing.

I want to serve underserved communities and do my share to ameliorate the health care crisis that our country faces. One evening as I shadowed a pediatric ER doctor, I was asked in Spanish, by several worried and uncomfortable parents, if I worked in the hospital. I replied that I was a student observing the doctor. Still they wanted to know if I would start working soon. ¡Le necesitamos aqui como doctora! We need you here as a doctor! The changing demographics of this country indicate the enormous need to address a variety of cultures in the delivery of health care. I would like to participate in the healing process by helping patients empower themselves. This caring transmission of information empowers the patient with knowledge. I consider it a privilege to be able to care for those in need of improved health. It should be a right, not a privilege, to see a doctor. Just as it is a right for me to speak to my congress person. Before interning in DC for a summer, I viewed congress people as powerful and distant entities. Whereas, now I believe that they are human beings whose job is to represent the public. I hope to be a representative of the medical field to those that are underserved; and, also become aware of the community's needs and function as a representative to affect policies which will address those needs.

Becoming a Physician

My decision to become a doctor is based on my commitment to serve as a primary care physician, where my interest in science and my compassion for humanity can be blended in order to communicate where I learn throughout my constant training. As a woman of color, I would like to be involved in the clinical environment so that I can help improve the quality of life for the patients whom I build relationships. As a socially responsible physician, I plan to dedicate myself to the recognition for the need for improvement in the quality of medicine for all.

Sample Essay #10

In light of the increase in highly qualified applicants and the resulting keen competition to fill a limited number of medical school slots, today's medical school applicant must stringently assess and scrutinize herself and know what it is she brings to the table. In this brief essay I will put on the table those things that make me an exceptional candidate for medical school as well as explain the inconsistencies in my academic record. It is my hope that what is presented will assist you in getting a sense of who this applicant is. Hopefully you will be able to look beyond the black and white of facts on paper and see a whole human being.

I attended a private, all Black, community school in Harlem. The girls went to school in the morning and the boys in the afternoon. When the school closed down due to funding and accreditation problems, I was forced to complete my high school training at Columbia University's high school equivalency program. In the Fall of that same year, I began college at Pace University. I was sixteen years old.

At sixteen, the independence of college life was a difficult adjustment. Having never attended school with anyone from a different race or gender made me ill-prepared for the relative freedom of post secondary education. With neither the maturity nor the preparation to be self-disciplined and self regulated, my grades suffered at the hands of my social development. Even though I had for two years in a row addressed the entering Freshman class of Pace University at their orientation, my grades spiraled downward. Eighteen credits short of graduating, I left school and entered the workforce.

Work experiences were mainly confined to the travel industry. I worked as a reservations and/ or ticketing agent for various airlines or as a sales representative for corporate travel agencies. These positions gave me the opportunity to travel frequently and extensively. I also worked as a newspaper advertising space sales representative. During my sales career, I joined The National Association of Professional Saleswomen and worked on the Executive Board as Director of Programming. I was the New York delegate at their 1988 National Convention and lead a sales seminar. My last position was as a reservations agent for Kuwait Airways. I was laid off while on vacation in India as a result of the Gulf War. I stayed in India and was invited to work on The Netraprakash Eye Camp organized by the Prasad Foundation.

Working in the Eye Camp proved to be the catalyst that brought together my desire to practice medicine with the maturity, self-confidence and perseverance I had acquired over the years. Some of my duties included coordinating patient traffic, assisting on post operative rounds and conducting patient interviews. When I returned to the States, I enrolled at The City College of New York. Aiming to improve my G.P.A., I took advanced level courses to qualify for a place in a Physician Assistant (PA) Program. While my applications were being reviewed by the four programs I'd applied to, I was selected as a mentee in The New York Coalition of 100 Black Women's Role Model Program I observed and worked with P.A.'s and M.D.'s in various health care settings and decided to direct my energies towards becoming a physician. So, when I received the acceptance letter from a P.A. Program, I declined the offer and continued my studies.

As a Howard Hughes research intern, I work in Dr. Patricia Broderick's pharmacology lab at The City University of New York Medical School and study the African plant ibogaine which may be used to treat cocaine addiction. Through in vivo electrochemistry and analysis of on-line production of neurotransmitters, we hope to find a dosage that avoids the ill-effect of cocaine withdrawal without becoming the new drug of choice. I have presented our work as a poster, published it as second author in The Society for Neuroscience Abstracts and plan to present it as a poster this Fall in Washington, D.C. at the Society's annual conference. I am a National Science Foundation sponsored chemistry workshop leader under the Alliance for Minority Participation Program. This summer I am a research intern in The Liver Center of The Albert Einstein College of Medicine. My project is to study the induction of cell differentiation due to retinoic acid.

While there were many diversions on my path, I believe the information presented along with my ever increasing desire to practice medicine make me an exceptional candidate for medical school.

Questions to Ask During the Medical School Interview

1. What special programs is the medical school noted for?

Academic Program
2. How is the school's curriculum set up in the preclinical and clinical years?
    A. Are there any special innovations?
    B. Are computers integrated into the curriculum?
    C. Is small group or problem based teaching integrated into the curriculum?
    D. Does the curriculum provide students with clinical exposure during the first two years?
3. How are students evaluated during the preclinical and clinical years?
4. Does the school provide its students with the opportunity to evaluate the curriculum?
    A. What recent changes have been made as a result of this feedback?
5. Does the school offer a note taking service or record its lectures?
6. How receptive are the faculty to student questions during and after lecture?
7. What opportunities are available for basic science or clinical research?
8. How many minority faculty are affiliated with the medical school?
    A. Are they involved in the basic science or clinical curriculum?
9. How well have minority students performed on the United States Medical Licensing Examination (USMLE) step I and II at your school?
    A. Does the school provide it students with a USMLE review program?
    B. How does the school assist students who do not pass?

Student Services
10. Does the school have a pre-matriculation program?
11. What kind of academic, personal, financial, and career counseling is available to students?
    A. Are these services offered to spouses?
12. Is there a minority student / faculty member mentor/advisor program?
13. Is there an office whose primary mission is to provide support to minority students?
    A. What specific services does this office provide?

Facilities
14. What are the high and low points of the facilities?
15. Are there computers available to students?
16. How many hospitals is the medical school affiliated with?
    A. Where are the hospitals located?
17. What type of clinical sites—ambulatory, private hospitals, rural settings -- are available for clerkships?
    A. Are rotations at other institutions or internationally allowed?

18. Is a car necessary?
>   A. Is parking a problem?

The Medical Student Body
19. What type of student does the medical school attract?
20. Do the minority students work together and support each other or is the atmosphere very individualistic and competitive?
21. How happy are the minority students with their medical school choice?
22. Is there an active minority medical student association (SNMA Chapter)?
23. Where do the minority medical students live?
>   A. How much does housing cost?
>   B. What is the cost of living?

Financial Aid
24. What are the current tuition and fees?
>   A. Is this expected to increase yearly? If so, at what rate?
25. Are there stable levels of federal financial aid and substantial amounts of university/medical school aid available to minority students?
26. Are there students who have an "unmet need" factored into their budget?
>   If so, where do the students come up with the extra funds?
27. Does the financial aid office actively look for fellowships and scholarships for it students?
28. Are spouses and dependents/children covered in a student's budget?
29. Is someone available to assist students with budgeting and financial planning?
30. Does the school provide guidance to its students on debt management?

Policies
31. Does the school have an established policy for situations of discrimination and a protocol of how that policy will be enforced?
>   A. Have there been any recent events in which this policy has been challenged?

Residency
32. May I see a list of residency programs and areas of medicine with which this school's recent minority graduates matched.

Endnote:
1. Organization of Student Representatives of the Association of American Medical Colleges. 30 Questions I Wish I Had Asked During My Medical School Interview. Washington, D.C. January, 1992.

Sample Interview Questions for Applicants

1. Why do you want to become a doctor?
2. What do you do in your spare time?
3. What are your specific goals in medicine?
4. What stimulated your interest in medicine?
5. Should equal access to medical services be a right of each citizen in the United States?
6. What do you intend to gain from a medical education?
7. Why do you think so many people want to become a doctor?
8. Pretend that our roles are reversed: what would you look for in an applicant?
9. There are 1,000 applicants equally as qualified as you. Why should we pick you?
10. What steps have you taken to acquaint yourself with what a doctor does?
11. What do you think is the most pressing issue in medicine today?
12. What would you do if you are not accepted into a medical school?
13. What are your positive qualities? Your negative qualities?
14. Describe your personality.
15. Do you have any unique skills or experiences that would bring value to our medical school?
16. Would you practice in an area where there is a shortage of physicians?
17. What aspect of medicine interests you the most?
18. What aspects of your life experiences do you think make you a good candidate for medical school?
19. Are your parents supportive of your goals?
20. Who has been the greatest role model in your life?
21. How do you cope with stress?
22. What do you like to do for fun?
23. How do you study?
24. What type of volunteer activities have you participated in?
25. Why do you think medicine is a rewarding profession?
26. What do you believe is the most stressful aspect of being a physician?
27. What are some of the biggest challenges physician face in the delivery of medical care?
28. How important is it for patients to be involved in the final decision making of their medical care?
29 Have you had any positive or negative experiences as a patient in a doctor's office or hospital?
30. Why did you apply to our medical school?
31. What resources or programs at our medical school do you look forward to utilizing the most?
32. What will be the most challenging aspect of medical school for you?
33. What have you done to prepare yourself for the rigors of medical school?
34. What do you feel is the most rewarding aspect of being a doctor?

Resource Information

Books

Inspirational

1. Drs. Sampson Davis, George Jenkins, Rameck Hunt, "**The Pact: Three Young Men Make a Promise and Fulfill a Dream.**" Riverhead Books 2002.
2. Drs. Sampson Davis, George Jenkins, Rameck Hunt, "**We Beat the Street: How a Friendship Led to Success.**" Dutton books 2005.
3. Ben Carson, MD, "**Gifted Hands: The Ben Carson Story.**" Zondervan Books 1990.
4. Ben Carson, MD, "**Think Big: Unleashing Your Potential for Excellence**." Zondervan Books 1992
5. Ben Carson, MD, "**The Big Picture**." Zondervan 2000.
6. Lori Arviso Alvord, MD, "**The Scalpel and the Silver Bear: The First Navajo Woman Surgeon Combines Western Medicine and Traditional Healing.**" Bantam 2000
7. Lewis Mehl-Madrona MD, "**Coyote Medicine: Lessons From Native American Healing.**" Touchstone 1998)
8. Yvonne S. Thornton, MD, "**The Ditchdigger's Daughters: A Black Family's Astonishing Success Story.**" Plume 1996.
9. Joan Cassell, "**The Woman in the Surgeons Body.**" Harvard University Press 2000.
10. Eliza Lo Chin, "**This Side of Doctoring: Reflections from Women in Medicine.**" Sage Publications 2001.
11. Donald Wilson, "**The Pride of African American History: Inventors, Scientists, Physicians, Engineers: Featuring Many Outstanding African Americans and More.**" Authorhouse 2003.

Medicine & Health Disparities

1. Paul Starr, "**The Social Transformation of American Medicine: The rise of a sovereign profession and the making of a vast industry.**" BasicBooks 1982.
2. David Satcher MD, Rubens J. Pamies MD, "**Multicultural Medicine and Health Disparities.**" McGraw-Hill Professional 2005.
3. Thomas LaVeist, "**Minority Populations and Health: An Introduction to Health Disparties in the U.S.**" Jossey-Bass 2005.
4. Thomas A. LaVeist, "**Race, Ethnicity, and Health: A Public Health Reader**" Jossey-Bass 2002.
5. Institute of Medicine, "**Unequal Treatment: Confronting Racial & Ethnic Disparities in Health.**" National Academies Press 2002.

Medical School Program Descriptions

1. Association of American Medical Colleges (AAMC), "**Medical School Admission's Requirements (MSAR)**"
2. Association of American Medical Colleges (AAMC) "**Minority Student Opportunities in United States Medical Schools.**"
3. "**U.S. News Ultimate Guide to Medical Schools**" Sourcebooks 2004

MCAT Preparation

1. James L. Flowers, Theodore Silvers, MD, "**Cracking the MCAT with Practice Questions on CD -ROM.**" Princeton Review 2004.
2. Rochelle Rothstein MD, "**Kaplan MCAT Comprehensive Review with CD-ROM 2005-2006.**" (Kaplan Mcat Premire Program).
3. Jonathan Orsay. "**Examkrackers McAt: Complete Study Package**" (Examkrackers) Osote Publishing 2003.

Application Essay

1. Emily Angel Baer, Stephanie B. Jones, "**Essays That Worked for Medical Schools: 40 Essays from Successful Applications to the Nation's Top Medical Schools.**" Ballantine Books 2003.
2. Dan Kaufman, Chris Dowhan, "**Essays That Will Get You into Medical School.**" Barron's Educational Series 2003.

Surviving The Medical School Years

1. Carmen Webb, "**Taking My Place in Medicine: A Guide for Minority Medical Students.**" Sage Publications 2000.

Summer Programs

A. Area Health Education Centers (AHEC) – National Office - http://bhpr.hrsa.gov/ahec/.

B. Summer Medical and Dental Education Program (SMDEP) - http://www.smdep.org/start.htm
    1. Case Western Reserve University School of Medicine (Cleveland, Ohio)
    2. Columbia University College of Physicians and Surgeons (New York City)
    3. David Geffen School of Medicine at UCLA (Los Angeles, CA)
    4. Duke University School of Medicine (Durham, NC)

B. Summer Medical and Dental Education Program (SMDEP) - http://www.smdep.org/start.htm
    5. Howard University Colleges of Arts and Sciences, Dentistry and Medicine (Wash., DC)
    6. The University of Texas Medical School at Houston (Houston, TX)
    7. UMDNJ – New Jersey Medical School (Newark, NJ)
    8. University of Louisville School of Medicine (Louisville, KY)
    9. University of Nebraska (Omaha, NE)
    10. University of Virginia School of Medicine (Charlottesville, VA)
    11. University of Washington School of Medicine (Seattle, WA)
    12. Yale University School of Medicine

C. Summer Undergraduate Research Programs via AAMC
            http://www.aamc.org/members/great/summerlinks.htm

D. Summer Program Database via AAMC
            http://services.aamc.org/summerprograms/GetProgs.cfm

E. There are many web pages listing summer programs. Some are updated better than others.
   Consider performing a web search using "minority pre-medical summer programs" or a related
   phrase.

Important Web Pages

High School Assessment Exams

ACT Assessment Exam – http://www.act.org/aap/
SAT exam - http://www.collegeboard.com/student/testing/sat/about.html

Historically Black Colleges and Universities

General List page - http://www.univsource.com/hbcu.htm

Postbaccalaureate Premedical programs

General List via AAMC - http://services.aamc.org/postbac/

Medical Schools

Allopathic Medical Schools - http://services.aamc.org/memberlistings/index.cfm
Osteopathic Medical Colleges - http://www.aacom.org/home-applicants/index.html
Duel degree programs - http://services.aamc.org/currdir/section3/degree2.cfm

Historically Black Medical Schools

Charles R. Drew University of Medicine and Science - http://www.cdrewu.edu/_022/_html/
Howard University College of Medicine - http://www.med.howard.edu/
Meharry Medical College - http://www.mmc.edu/
Morehouse School of Medicine - http://www.msm.edu/

Medical College Admissions Test (MCAT)

Registration - www.aamc.org/mcat
Scores for non-AMCAS participating schools- http://services.aamc.org/mcatthx
Fee reduction program - http://www.aamc.org/students/applying/fap/
Practice exams (click under browse a topic MCAT) - www.aamc.org/publications/start.htm
MCAT Practice on-line - www.e-mcat.com
The Princeton Review - www.princetonreview.com
The Stanley Kaplan - www.kaptest.com

Medical School Applications & Admissions

AMCAS application - http://www.aamc.org/students/amcas/start.htm
AACOMAS application - https://aacomas.aacom.org/
Early Decision Information - http://www.aamc.org/students/applying/programs/earlydecision.htm
The Medical Minority Applicant Registry (Med - MAR)
        http://www.aamc.org/students/minorities/resources/medmar.htm

Financing the Medical Education

Free Application for Federal Student Aid – www.fafsa.ed.gov
MEDLOANS - http://www.aamc.org/students/medloans/start.htm
National Medical Fellowships - http://www.nmfonline.org/index.html
Financial Aid Information via AAMC - http://www.aamc.org/students/financing/start.htm
Financial Planning via AAMC - http://www.aamc.org/students/financing/md2/start.htm

Government Scholarship Programs

National Health Service Corps - http://nhsc.bhpr.hrsa.gov/
Army Health Corps - http://www.goarmy.com/amedd/
Air force Health Careers - http://www.airforce.com
Navy Health Careers - http://www.navy.com/healthcare/physicians

Careers in Medicine

AAMC Careers in Medicine - http://www.aamc.org/students/cim/specialties.htm
Anesthesiology - www.asahq.org/
Dermatology - www.aad.org
Emergency Medicine - http://www.acep.org/
Family Medicine - www.aafp.org
General Surgery - http://www.facs.org
Geriatric Medicine - http://www.americangeriatrics.org/
Internal Medicine - http://www.doctorsforadults.com/index.html
Obstetrics and Gynecology - http://www.acog.org/
Ophthalmology - http://www.aao.org/
Orthopedics - http://www.aaos.org/
Pediatrics - www.aap.org
Physical Medicine and Rehabilitation - http://www.aapmr.org/
Psychiatry - http://www.psych.org/
Radiology - www.acr.org/

Medical Student and Professional Medical Associations

Association of American Indian Physicians (AAIP) - http://www.aaip.com/
Inter- American College of Physicians and Surgeons - http://www.icps.org/main.htm
National Hispanic Medical Association (NHMA) - www.nhmamd.org
National Medical Association (NMA) - http://www.nmanet.org
The Student National Medical Association (SNMA) - www.snma.org
Latino Medical Student Association (LMSA) - http://www.lmsa.net/
National Network of Latin American Med. Students (NNLAMS) - www.nnlams.com
National Boricua Latino Health Organization - http://nblho.org/
Association of Native American Medical Students (ANAMS) - http://www.aaip.com
American Medical Student Association - http://www.amsa.org/

Now It's Your Turn To Write The Pages of History